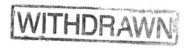

BETTER CANCER CARE

Also of interest to readers of this volume are selected titles in the publisher's series:
POLICY AND PRACTICE IN HEALTH AND SOCIAL CARE

2: Charlotte Pearson (ed.), *Direct Payments and Personalisation of Care* (2006)

3: Joyce Cavaye, *Hidden Carers* (2006)

4: Mo McPhail (ed.), *Service User and Carer Involvement: Beyond Good Intentions* (2007)

6: Alison Petch, *Health and Social Care: Establishing a Joint Future?* (2007)

10: Rebecca L. Jones and Richard Ward (eds.), *LGBT Issues: Looking Beyond Categories* (2009)

11: Jacqueline H. Watts, *Death, Dying and Bereavement: Issues for Practice* (2009)

BETTER CANCER CARE
A Systemic Approach to Practice

Liz Forbat, Gill Hubbard and Nora Kearney

DUNEDIN ACADEMIC PRESS
Edinburgh

Published by
Dunedin Academic Press Ltd
Hudson House
8 Albany Street
Edinburgh EH1 3QB
Scotland

ISBN 978-1-906716-09-7

British Library Cataloguing in Publication Data
A catalogue record for this book is available from the British Library

Typeset by Makar Publishing Production
Printed and bound in the UK by Cromwell Press Group
Printed on paper from sustainable resources

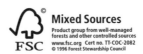

Mixed Sources
Product group from well-managed
forests and other controlled sources
www.fsc.org Cert no. TT-COC-2082
FSC © 1996 Forest Stewardship Council

Contents

Acknowledgements

The data that is used in this book is drawn from a study in which a large number of people with cancer, their partners and healthcare professionals participated. Thanks go, primarily, to those who spoke about their experiences of cancer with the research team.

We also wish to thank the following people for their role in the project who were involved in data collection, study design and research support: Bridgeen Duffy, Nicola Illingworth, Aileen Ireland, Maureen James, Ruth Jepson, Lucy Johnston, Kate Knighting, Neneh Rowa-Dewar, Sara Walker, Mike Wilson and Allison Worth. People affected by cancer also contributed to the design of the research: our thanks go to them in their role as advisors to the Cancer Care Research Centre.

Thanks also go to our two critical readers of the manuscript: Caroline Cochrane and Marian Gerry. Remaining errors are ours, of course, not theirs.

The research study, from which this book draws its data, was funded by the Scottish Government. The opinions expressed within reflect the views of the authors, not the funders.

Preface

At its core, this book proposes one message: the experience of cancer affects not just individuals. Although the disease resides in individuals, the effects of it are felt across far reaching contexts and multiple relationships. The family, work colleagues and health and social care professionals can be considered both resources and recipients of the impact of a serious diagnosis. For example, family dynamics and family functioning will play a part in how the disease is related to and the overall (ill) health experience. Traditionally, cancer care practice and policy have failed to address these, focusing either on the disease, or, at best, on the individual who has the cancer.

Writing a book about cancer which adopts an approach explicitly locating cancer in its social and personal milieu came about due to the increasing recognition that people's experiences of health are mediated by context. One of the core lines of argument in this book is that to provide cancer care and to understand the experience of cancer one must understand this context in its widest sense. Consequently, we felt it appropriate to position ourselves explicitly in relation to this, and provide readers with an understanding of the wider systems that inform our thinking and contributions to this book.

I (LF) am a research psychologist with over ten years of experience working in fields associated with families and ill health. I was working in health research when I was diagnosed with cancer in 2003. Seeking to connect up my professional life with my experience of cancer, I sought out a research post at the Cancer Care Research Centre (CCRC), University of Stirling. Working at CCRC enabled me to use my energies to contribute to improving cancer care by encouraging less emphasis on hospital systems and more on the people undergoing treatment and those around them. Alongside my research experience I have undertaken training in family therapy and systemic practice. It is that theoretical lens, and approach to practice, that is woven throughout this book by locating people affected by cancer in the context of their relationships and wider socio–cultural spaces.

I (GH) am a sociologist with ten years research experience in health and illness. I project managed the study upon which this book is based. Overall, the study highlighted the importance of locating people's experiences of cancer within social contexts. It was during the study that my partner, who was only forty-eight years old at the time, had a heart attack. This personal and direct experience of living with a partner who had had a heart attack brought it home only too clearly how family members collectively respond to, and manage, illness. My partner made a fantastic recovery, and is probably much healthier, and certainly much fitter, post-heart attack. This personal experience informed the way in which I understand people's experiences of health and illness, including cancer.

I (NK) am a cancer nurse with over twenty-five years experience in cancer care and seventeen years in cancer care research. I was the principal investigator for the study from which this book draws its data. I set up the CCRC in 2003 with the aim of working in partnership with people affected by cancer to undertake research that would improve clinical care. My experience as a cancer nurse allowed me significant insight into the complexities of people's experiences and how this affected their response to illness; this was reinforced when my mother died of lung cancer.

We would like to thank all the people affected by cancer who participated in the interviews on which this book is based. Their generosity of time and energy means that this book is able to pursue the goal of contributing to a sea change in how people affected by cancer are supported by services. We hope we have done them justice.

Chapter 1

Introduction

This book reports on research that sought to contribute to the development of Scottish cancer services, with a particular focus on improving patient and carer experiences. The study included explicit aims to explore the experiences of people affected by cancer in the first year following diagnosis.

The research recruited sixty-six people newly diagnosed with one of the most frequently occurring cancers in Scotland, namely breast, prostate, lung, colorectal and gynaecological cancers. These individuals participated in a series of prospective interviews over the course of the first year following their diagnosis. Each individual was asked to identify someone who shared closely in their experience (typically a relative/friend) and a healthcare professional (typically a nurse), who was then invited to participate in interviews. This produced the largest qualitative data-set of its kind in mapping people's experiences of cancer care in Scotland. It led to a reconceptualisation of cancer care and cancer experience: a whole-systems and relational approach to cancer, which is described and illustrated in detail in this book. Although the data comes from a study on cancer, readers interested in other areas of chronic illness will find resonance with the ideas and practice implications that are developed.

This introduction outlines the theoretical framework and summarises the policy context in which the research and people's experiences of cancer care are situated, before outlining the content of subsequent chapters.

A systemic approach to cancer care

This book seeks to reposition thinking, practice and policy about cancer and cancer care. It is an explicitly ambitious and extravagant attempt to reframe thinking about *what it means to have cancer* and *what it means to work in cancer care*. We grapple with some of the challenges that present themselves to people affected by cancer, placing them at the centre of this reconceptualisation of cancer care.

A mild assertion resides in policy and literature that other individuals are also connected with experiences of ill health, primarily through the construction of the 'carer' identity and role. We use the term *mild* advisedly – and not to contest the important role that unpaid carers hold, nor the services which have sought to support them. Rather, we wish to assert that the separation of the person providing care and the person receiving care serves to treat them as individuals and neglects to understand them, and their interactions, in relationship with each other (Forbat, 2005) and results in 'reproducing a false dichotomy between carers and carees' (Forbat, 2003: 68). In this book, we use the term 'partner' when referring to someone who shares closely in the experience of the cancer. This may be a spouse, or another relative such as an adult child or friend. The term 'carer' is only maintained when this is the term used by the individual themselves during the course of the conversation. When the exact nature of the relationship is salient (for example discussing mother–daughter relationships), then the speaker is identified more specifically. We use the phrase 'people affected by cancer' to identify the individual with the disease and the people around them who they deem to be impacted upon by the cancer. 'People affected by cancer' has to include people beyond just the cancer patient.

Alongside the proliferation of carer literature and policy there has been the adoption of the term 'whole system approach' within policy of late. It latches onto the drive for joined-up working between governmental departments such as social care, housing, health care and benefits. Systems theory has been applied in community action research to progress such partnership working (Burns, 2007). This adoption of partnership working, or whole system approach, has heralded organisational adaptations (new services, different communications between silos of governmental departments). We believe these shifts signal a growing recognition of individual and organisational connectivity – of the importance of interrelationships. It is this notion that we seek to nurture and develop in this book, to illustrate how such ideas can evolve into better cancer care.

The way in which we use 'whole systems' in this book, and our proposal for a broader and more valuable use of the term for understanding patient experience, is necessarily somewhat different to its application within policy and government. The way we approach 'carers' also necessarily moves to a much wider approach to considering the entire system/networks that are affected by and mediate the illness.

Our approach stems from the use of whole system working as applied within disciplines such as family therapy. In short, 'system' refers to a wide network of people who are connected to the person with the disease. We refer to this as a systemic approach. This immediately extends the description beyond that used within policy and away from a purely organisational definition. The system can be conceived as a sequence of different environments, such as family (close and extended), friends, schools, workplaces, communities and leisure facilities. For example, for people who are in paid employment, their workplace is one social context that has a bearing on how cancer is experienced.

Larger contextual influences also play their part, such as the cultural environs including the socio-historical space in which cancer is experienced. Improvements in screening and treatments have led to increased survival from many cancers. The term 'cancer survivor' is increasingly being used in UK policy and builds an expectation that people will not die of the disease. Following the commitment in the *Cancer Reform Strategy* (Department of Health, 2007) to improve patients' experience of living with and beyond cancer, a National Cancer Survivorship Initiative was established. In Scotland, arising from *Better Cancer Care* (Scottish Government, 2008), a Living with Cancer working group, which is part of the Scottish Cancer Taskforce, was launched. One of the outcomes of these policy drives is in reframing what it means to live with and beyond cancer and informs practitioner views of patients moving beyond active treatment.

However, despite treatment changes and policy, for some people cancer will be a fatal disease (Costain-Schou and Hewison, 1999). Further, media portrayals of high profile people who die from cancer can affirm the belief that cancer is a death sentence. This magnifies established social beliefs about the fatality of cancer. People's relationship with the disease is therefore based on this dialectic of survivorship and fatality.

Connected to each of these contexts is the collective and shared language with which people describe their experiences of cancer. The systemic approach is mindful of constructivist understandings of language, and the recursive connections between language and meaning, located in time and place. That is, an appreciation of the importance of how people talk about experiences is active in constructing meaning.

The systemic model is based on the idea that individuals (and the problems they live with) cannot and should not be understood in isolation (Burnham, 1986). A further key assumption is that linear models of cause and effect do not accurately reflect the lived complexities of a diagnosis such as cancer. As we argue throughout this book, cancer may impact upon relationships, relationships impact on cancer, and each of these recursively and iteratively connect with wider social and cultural understandings of, and responses to, the disease. Fundamentally, there is a need to understand the entire context in which people experience and make sense of their illness, and particularly their interconnectedness and interrelationships with others. In the case of cancer, this means broadening out from a patient-centred approach to embracing the wider context in which the illness is experienced, including the relational and social aspects and impacts of cancer and cancer care. In so doing, a broader and more developed definition of whole system working is invoked and warranted.

Although the adoption of patient-centred approaches have doubtlessly improved the way in which services respond to people with cancer (and other diseases), it is predicated upon an assumption that illnesses are experienced solely by individuals. We know from research evidence that this is not how illness is experienced. For example, when someone has a health condition that has clear links to food and nutrition, an entire family's way of life and way of eating may be impacted upon. A study investigating coeliac's disease and heart disease illustrated this family-wide behavioural effect with clarity (Gregory, 2005). Likewise, when someone is diagnosed with an hereditary or communicable disease, it is understandable that other members of the family and wider networks may consider the impact of that diagnosis on themselves. For example, the diagnosis of a parent with dementia may trigger concerns about its occurrence in later generations and impacts upon help-seeking behaviour and screening uptake (Corner and Bond, 2004; Gershenson Hodgson *et al.*, 1999). Thus, adopting an explicitly relational approach to cancer is likely to highlight important features of the experience that have hitherto been marginalised by the overemphasis on individuals and disease processes.

Critically, the systemic approach adopted within this book prioritises a relational and contextual understanding of cancer, recognising and acting upon an assertion that the impact of cancer is far wider than the individual with the disease.

Policy context

This study took place in post-devolution Scotland, where wider health and specifically cancer-related policy was regarded as a top priority, often in the media spotlight. The study's findings are situated within these policy directives but are also contextualised with reference to wider bodies of policy and thought, from England and beyond. The purpose of this section is to give an overview of the policy context rather than a critique. We have selected the policy that sets the trends for service delivery in cancer care, focusing on patient involvement, shifting the balance of care, the culture of care and the role of informal carers.

In 2001, the Scottish Executive cancer strategy, *Cancer in Scotland: Action for Change,* was launched (Scottish Executive, 2001a). It did not prescribe actions plans but rather set the scene, which at the time was focused on cancer prevention, reducing waiting times and delays for treatment, and the introduction of Regional Cancer Advisory Groups and Managed Clinical Networks as vehicles for greater integration. It recognised that more people will be living with cancer, thus requiring support services and information to meet their needs. It acknowledged the role of primary care teams as key to providing care since most people with cancer spend the majority of their time in the community and not in hospital, and made passing reference to the significance of rehabilitation services and clinical psychology. A number of challenges for cancer services were raised including the limitations of health professionals' time for talking to people with cancer to help them understand their diagnosis and all its implications; having to give a delayed and unexpected diagnosis of cancer because symptoms did not immediately suggest cancer; palliative care remaining an untapped resource due to its association with death and dying; the limited resource effort available to manage the transition of people with cancer between primary and secondary care; and the uneven quality and quantity of information provided to people with cancer.

Putting patients at the centre of quality improvement and frameworks so that services are designed round the needs of patients and securing better outcomes for patients became a key theme for the second phase of the cancer strategy (Scottish Executive, 2004). This agenda of involving and placing the experience of patients with cancer at the centre of service organisation and delivery was emphasised in the Calman–Hine Report (1995) and has gained momentum during the last few years through projects like the Cancer Partnership Project, a three-year project funded by Macmillan Cancer Relief and the Department of Health aimed at promoting user involvement activity in all cancer networks in England (Sitzia *et al.*, 2004) and a three-year project funded by the Scottish Executive, Developing cancer services: Patient and carer experiences (from which this research arose).

At the time of writing this book *Better Cancer Care: An Action Plan* was published (Scottish Government, 2008), progressing the policy agenda for services in Scotland. Prevention and detection were presented here as individual responsibilities set against a backdrop of population-based statistics/epidemiology. Survivorship – living with and beyond cancer – forms an important new direction for cancer policy indicating the need to continue to provide services for people following active treatment.

Several themes in this book – patient involvement and self-care, partnership working and community-based care, a culture of caring, the role of partners/carers – are also highlighted in other Scottish health and cancer policy, and are discussed briefly below to set further context for the data that follows.

Patient involvement and self care

Better Cancer Care (Scottish Government, 2008) reaffirms the policy agenda of patient and public involvement and focuses on involvement in healthcare policy, planning and care practice (Hubbard *et al.*, 2007), in the context of ongoing conceptual tensions (Forbat *et al.*, 2009). The study on which this book is based coincided with the implementation of key health policy documents including *A National Framework for Service Change in the NHS in Scotland* (Scottish Executive, 2005a). Its vision of the future includes building a health service that starts from the patient experience, engages the public, and involves patients in their own care. Further associated action plans relating to patient involvement were also published at the time the study was conducted including *Delivering Care, Enabling Health* (Scottish Executive, 2006a), which sets out an action plan for nursing, midwifery and allied health professions. It emphasises that patients should be regarded as partners rather than passive recipients of care. *Partnership for Care* (Scottish Executive, 2003) and, most recently, *Co-ordinated, Integrated and Fit for Purpose* (Scottish Executive, 2007) echo the policy context outlined in *Delivering for Health* (Scottish Executive, 2005b) by recommending an ethos of enablement and self-managed care with people and their carers taking greater control. Patient involvement in decision-making works in conjunction with self-care, which is defined by the Scottish Executive (2005a: 68) as 'the individual taking action to maintain health, prevent illness, seek and adhere to treatment, manage symptoms and side effects, accomplish recovery and rehabilitation and cope with chronic illness and disability. Engagement in self-care facilitates a partnership between health service users, their carers and health professionals to ensure optimal health outcomes'.

The emphasis on self-management or self-care within English health policy has aimed to promote greater involvement of people in the management of long-term or chronic conditions such as cancer, and firm support for self-care can be found in a number of additional Department of Health policy documents including *The NHS Plan* (Department of Health, 2000); *The Expert Patient* (Department of Health, 2001); *Supporting People with Long Term Conditions* (Department of Health, 2005a); *Self Care – a Real Choice* (Department of Health, 2005b) and *Our Health, Our Care, Our Say* (Department of Health, 2006). Such policy reports reflect moves towards greater patient involvement in health care generally, and decision-making and management of their own care specifically, moving away from the traditional top-down 'doctor knows best' model of care to a culture where patients' experiences and contributions to their own care are considered essential to meeting their health care needs.

Shifting the balance of care

At the time of carrying out the study, the Scottish Government (then the Scottish Executive) called for greater partnership working and care in local communities. An aim of the policy agenda for partnership is to provide seamless care and bridge any gaps between primary and acute sectors. Policy related to the management of long-term conditions, for instance, emphasises that care depends on both community and outpatient-based care to support self-care and on partnership working between community and hospital care (Scottish Executive, 2005a). *A National Framework for Service Change in the NHS in Scotland,* (Scottish Executive, 2005a) states that healthcare services should be delivered predominantly in local communities and be coordinated by primary care, operating within an integrated National Health Service (NHS) collaborating with other partners. Traditional ways of delivering care are rejected and replaced by new ways of working including a proposal to seek alternatives to consultant-led, hospital-based follow-up care. This framework also states that patients want access to local high-quality services as quickly as possible and delivered by a suitably trained professional.

A key focus of policy is care in local communities. *Delivering for Health* (Scottish Executive, 2005b) was a key document when this study was conducted. It describes the main actions to implement the recommendations of the *National Framework for Service Change* (Scottish Executive, 2005c) and highlights the changes that patients will see, including more health care being provided locally in general practitioner

(GP) practices and carers being treated as partners in the provision of care. *Co-ordinated, Integrated and Fit for Purpose* (Scottish Executive, 2007) provides strategic direction to health and social care services and practitioners who deliver rehabilitation services. It also recommends local service provision with a strong community focus, improved access and smooth transitions between primary and secondary care services, multidisciplinary teams and multiagency partnerships. A review of nursing in the community in Scotland (Scottish Executive, 2006b) reaffirms a shift towards multidisciplinary and multiagency teams, self-care and local community provision. It proposes a single point of contact for all nursing services – community health nursing – so that people are not confused about which service or nurse to approach and emphasises the important role that nurses play in co-ordinating and organising care provided by other professions and agencies for people they care for. More recently, *Better Cancer Care* (Scottish Government, 2008: 79) suggests a shift in care through 'improving communication to patients and between professional disciplines and services'.

At the time of writing this book, this policy emphasis was developed further by the Scottish Government (2009): 'By Shifting the Balance of Care (SBC) we aim to improve the health and wellbeing of the people of Scotland by increasing our emphasis on health improvement and anticipatory care, providing more continuous care and more support closer to home. This requires a partnership approach between the NHS, local authorities and the third sector.'

The importance of partnership working was at the forefront of policy when the study was carried out, for example, in England with the White Paper *Our Health, Our Care, Our Say* (Department of Health, 2006). This paper highlights the need for local authorities and NHS organisations to operate with shared agendas and develop strong working relationships if they are to deliver the government's vision of maximising choice for service users, as well as providing more individualised packages of care and support. The NHS Quality Improvement in Scotland (QIS, 2007) and the National Institute of Health and Clinical Excellence guidelines (2004) also emphasise the importance of other services and sectors in healthcare planning and service delivery, including social care. The policy reinforces the need for services to extend their partnerships to include service users and also consolidates the place of independent providers in the health and social care market. Although Scottish and English health policy has similarities, it is argued that Scotland places greater emphasis on partnership working between different NHS sectors and the NHS and other organisations, whereas England has a more market driven agenda involving the private sector (Greer and Rowland, 2008). More recently, the Darzi report (2008) reinforces the empowerment of patient choice.

Culture of caring

Central in much health and cancer care policy is the importance of delivering services within a culture of caring. For example, *Delivering Care, Enabling Health* (Scottish Executive, 2006a), sets out an action plan for nursing, midwifery and allied health professions (NMAHPs) emphasising that at the heart of good nursing is 'caring', which is defined as 'seeing the human being – not the patient number' (2006a: 3); a vision also reinforced through current NHS QIS (2007) standards. The plan claims that NMAHPs are champions of the patient's experience and places a culture of caring with the following attributes – approachability, kindness, courtesy, empathy and an ability to listen respectfully to the person – at the heart of good NMAHP practice. Moreover, the importance of communication as a key element of a culture of caring is emphasised in *Cancer in Scotland. Action for Change. A Guide to Securing Access to Information*, which states that 'All staff concerned with patient care should be aware of potential problems with communication and be aware that patients often find it difficult to take in information during consultations, especially just after hearing a diagnosis of cancer or other "bad news"' (Scottish Executive, 2001b: 10).

Role of unpaid carers

The term 'unpaid carer' is used to describe individuals who care for a friend, relative or neighbour without receiving paid income other than that received through the welfare/benefits system (Office for Public Management (OPM) *et al.*, 2006). Unpaid carers are the largest group of care providers in Scotland and, as such, are the biggest section of the Scottish care 'workforce', making a significant contribution to society in both fiscal and pragmatic terms (Carers UK, 2002; OPM *et al.*, 2006). The Scottish Government's health policy calls for greater empowerment of patients and carers and greater collaboration between them and health and social care organisations. Unpaid carers are central to the core strategic health policies of providing more community and home-based care and reducing hospital admissions (Information Services Division (ISD), 2006; Scottish Executive, 2005b; Scottish Executive, 2005d). Carers also have a role in supporting self-care in the community (Scottish Executive, 2005b; Scottish Executive, 2005d). Indeed, *Delivering for Health* underlines the role carers play in supporting patient self-care, focusing on a call to determine carers' perceptions of this role to ensure that patients and carers have the necessary skills and knowledge, as well as an appropriate person to contact for further support if required (Scottish Executive, 2005b).

The 'caring relationship' is recognised in *A National Framework for Service Change in the NHS in Scotland*, (Scottish Executive, 2005a), which refers to the *Community Care and Health (Scotland) Act* (Scottish Executive Health Department, 2002), which places a legislative duty on NHS Boards to support carers through the development of local NHS Carer Information Strategies. In addition, *Delivering for Health* (Scottish

Executive, 2005b) highlights that carers will be treated as partners in the provision of care and *Co-ordinated, Integrated and Fit for Purpose* (Scottish Executive, 2007) echoes the policy directive outlined in *Delivering for Health* by recommending an ethos of enablement and self-managed care with people and their carers taking greater control. Similarly, in England, NICE (2004) guidelines recognise the central role of relatives and other carers in supporting patients.

Recent policy (Scottish Government, 2008) makes an explicit assumption about the role of carers in the context of patient care. Specific ideas of two-way communication between healthcare professionals and people affected by cancer, treatment decision-making and self-care all acknowledge that informal carers have a role.

Structure of the book

The book consists of ten chapters. Chapter 1, this introduction, outlines the systemic approach that informs the analysis and findings presented in this book. The policy context is described to position the study in the wider political and practice documentation.

Chapter 2 describes the methods used to conduct the study. This includes a description of the people affected by cancer and healthcare professionals involved in the study, how they were identified and recruited, a description of the interviews that were conducted and analytical strategy.

The main body of the book presents people's experiences of cancer by applying a systemic approach. Quotations and examples from research interviews with people affected by cancer and people working in cancer care have been carefully selected to illuminate a particular aspect of a concept or issue. The focus is on the experiences of people affected by cancer, their relationships and the contexts of their lives. Each chapter draws explicitly on the idea of cancer as a disease that is experienced in relation to others in social contexts.

Chapter 3 outlines the family context for making sense of the experience of cancer. The role of different family members and the changes in relationships that occur when someone develops cancer build an argument regarding the joint ownership, management and impact of cancer within families. Thus the systemic approach asserts that a change to one part of a system (for example, the diagnosis of cancer to an individual in the family) impacts upon all other parts of the system (relationships and roles will alter and shift). Cancer is positioned as a family affair.

Chapter 4 describes patient and partner relationships with professionals, including those in the community and acute sectors. This chapter builds upon the idea of relationships developed in Chapter 3, but extends this to professionals, and how these impact upon the experience of cancer. This underlines the value placed on relationships between people affected by cancer and the professionals in the context of hospital and community care services.

Chapter 5 highlights the importance of relationships beyond the immediate family and professional networks; it draws attention to the relationships between people with a cancer diagnosis. This experiential interconnectivity demonstrates how cancer is related to and mediates relationships with other people. Thus, a systemic approach focuses not only on relationships between people, but relationships with the illness.

Chapter 6 continues to explore the role of relationships. It focuses on employment, employers and colleagues. Further, it draws attention to a key source of purpose and identity, that is, people's relationship with work itself. This wider social location of cancer provides an opportunity to further elaborate the systemic approach, moving beyond the disease model and into an understanding of the varied contexts that organise identity.

Chapter 7 continues the exploration begun in the previous chapter, regarding the extent to which cancer forces a disruption to, and/or an integration of cancer into, identity. Cancer becomes a dominant context in which identity work is performed, and where people reflect and reassess their past, present and future sense of self. This is built upon systemic understandings of self, which view differing contexts, in this example the diagnosis of cancer, as creating opportunities for dynamically changing identities.

Chapter 8 focuses on the physicality of cancer, including elaborating on the identity implications of a physical illness that were discussed in the previous chapter. Drawing on accounts of symptoms, treatment and investigations, this chapter looks at how people with cancer relate to their bodies and how others, notably healthcare professionals, relate to the physical sequelae of cancer. This builds a case for locating symptoms and side-effects and situating the physical presence of cancer in the context of people's lives.

Chapter 9 takes a much broader focus, by looking at the dominant cultural and social contexts and how these impact on and mediate experiences of cancer. The socio-historical and personal contexts in which the person experiences cancer gives meaning to the experience, which is essential for better cancer care.

The final chapter outlines the systemic approach to achieving better cancer care by drawing on the research data, and presents a conceptual discussion and synthesis of the main findings.

Chapter 2

Methods: research methods, procedure and sample

This book is based on a qualitative study conducted over a period of eighteen months. Three serial, longitudinal semi-structured interviews with people diagnosed with cancer were carried out over the course of a year following diagnosis. A partner and healthcare professional nominated by the individual with cancer were also interviewed.

The aim of the project was to explore the experiences of people affected by cancer in the first year following diagnosis in Scotland. NHS ethical approval was gained via the Central Office for Research Ethics Committees (COREC), and local research and development approval was obtained in the four clinical sites where people affected by cancer and healthcare professionals were recruited. All people involved in the study gave written informed consent and had the right to withdraw from the study at any time for any reason. Personal data recorded on all documentation relating to the study was regarded as confidential. Each of the extracts drawn upon in this book have had all identifying details altered to preserve participants' anonymity.

Clinical sites

The study took place across four of the largest health boards in Scotland. Three nurse consultants and one manager within each site provided access to consultants and/or cancer nurse specialists, to facilitate recruitment of people affected by cancer to the study.

Sampling and recruitment

Sixty-six people diagnosed with cancer were recruited to the study. The focus on the most frequent diagnoses resulted in the study exploring adult's experiences of cancer. The sample included eighteen people with colorectal cancer, twelve women with breast cancer, nine women with gynaecological cancer, seventeen people with lung cancer and ten men with prostate cancer. Purposive sampling was used to ensure that experiences of cancer were explored through the perspectives of people with different socio-demographic characteristics. This sampling strategy was not designed to derive a representative sample but to enable the researchers to understand experiences of cancer and cancer care from a diverse group including:

- males (thirty-five) and females (thirty-one) with cancer;
- people living in rural (sixteen) and urban (fifty) areas;
- people of different ages (just over a third were aged between thirty-one and sixty years old and the remainder were sixty-one years old or over).

A conscious effort was made to include people from different ethnic minority groups. However, this was unsuccessful as only very small numbers of people from these groups were diagnosed with cancer during the period of recruitment in the cancer centres where healthcare professionals were recruiting for the study, and none consented to participate.

Inclusion criteria ensured that participants were adults over the age of sixteen years, able to give informed consent and were diagnosed with one of the following cancers: breast, lung, colorectal, prostate or gynaecological cancers. A final criterion was that this must also be the person's first diagnosis of cancer.

Recruitment

People with cancer were recruited through outpatient clinics within approximately six weeks following diagnosis. Recruitment took place in the winter of 2005 to early spring 2006. Working within ethical guidelines, researchers were not the first point of contact for people with cancer regarding the study. The initial approach to potential participants was by local clinicians. They briefly outlined the study and provided them with an information letter and information sheet. The clinicians asked the people with cancer if they were willing to be contacted by the researchers who would provide them with more information. Upon the request of local clinicians, the researchers attended the clinic area, to supply more information about the study after the consultation if people with cancer wished to discuss the study. The researcher either spoke to the person with cancer in the clinic or telephoned them to provide more information, and confirmed willingness to participate and arranged to visit for the first interview.

Sample and recruitment of partners

Each person with cancer recruited to the study was asked by the researcher before the first interview to identify a family member or close friend who also knew about their experiences. Primarily these people were partners, and are referred to as such in subsequent chapters rather than as 'carers'. At times, patients nominated other relatives, such as daughters, and this relationship is marked as such in the quotations used. Those nominated were asked if they were willing to take part in the study. Only those who gave written informed consent were included. Forty-three partners were nominated who all consented to take part and were included in the study.

Sampling and recruitment of healthcare professionals

Each person with cancer recruited to the study was asked by the researcher during the first interview to identify a healthcare professional who knew about their experiences. Those nominated were asked if they were willing to take part in the study. Only those who gave written informed consent were included. Forty-two healthcare professionals were nominated, twenty-six of whom consented to take part and twenty were interviewed. A failure to nominate partly indicated that within the first few months of receiving a diagnosis patients had not established relationships with healthcare professionals. Alongside this was a lack of willingness to consent to take part in the study on the part of healthcare professionals; rationales presented to researchers suggested that they do not feel as though they possess sufficient in-depth knowledge about the experiences of the patient within their first few months of diagnosis. Additionally, professionals mentioned the pressure of work and the fact that participation in this particular study was not a priority for them.

Interviews

Semi-structured interviews were designed to capture key experiences in the first year following diagnosis. The interviews were audio-recorded with participants' consent and transcribed. The rationale for when each interview took place focused on key episodes of the cancer experience and care provision in the first year following diagnosis. These were:

- *Experiences of symptoms prior to diagnosis and being told the diagnosis.* An interview within approximately 6 weeks of being told the diagnosis was scheduled so that people with cancer could discuss their experiences occurring at the initial stage of their illness.

- *Experiences of the first course of treatments including surgery, chemotherapy, radiotherapy.* An interview between 4 and 6 months of being told the diagnosis was scheduled so that people with cancer could relate their experiences occurring during treatment.

- *Experiences of follow-up and after care.* An interview between 8 and 9 months of being told the diagnosis was scheduled so that people with cancer could relate their experiences of the end of treatment and reflections on follow-up care and living with cancer in the longer term.

Most people with cancer took part in the first interviews within 6 weeks following diagnosis, with the exception of nine people with cancer who were interviewed within ten weeks of diagnosis. Most people with cancer took part in the second interviews within four and six months following diagnosis, with the exception of some people with lung cancer who were interviewed slightly earlier, owing to the likely poorer prognosis and a desire to capture their experiences as they received treatment. Half of the people with cancer were interviewed for the third time between eight and ten months following diagnosis and approximately half were interviewed between ten and fourteen months following diagnosis (only three people with cancer were interviewed after twelve months). Table 2.1 shows the number of people interviewed at each stage. Ten people with cancer withdrew from the study and four people died.

Table 2.1 Number of patients and partners interviewed

Interview	N
Interview 1	
Patient only	29
Joint patient and partner	37
Partner only	6
Total	72
Interview 2	
Patient only	32
Joint patient and partner	26
Partner only	5
Total	63
Interview 3	
Patient only	27
Joint patient and partner	25
Partner only	5
Total	57
Overall total	**192**

At the start of the study it was made clear to participants that they could withdraw without giving a reason and without it affecting their care, thus, it is not possible to identify why some people withdrew and did participate in a second or third interview. Prospective interviews allowed for the building of accounts across time, rather than adopting a cross-sectional approach, which would not allow for each of the participants' accounts to progress between research encounters. This prospective, longitudinal method has been positioned as one which fits well with a systemic approach to understanding illness (Rolland, 1994).

Individual and dyadic interviews

People with cancer were given the choice of being interviewed on their own or accompanied by their nominated partner. The choice was left with participants, to provide them with as much control over the interview situation as possible. Some partners were present during the interview with the individual but were also interviewed on their own. There are advantages and disadvantages of conducting joint interviews (Morris, 2001). A potential disadvantage is that people may not wish to talk about certain experiences or worries in the presence of their partner. However, this is balanced by a potential advantage of people reflecting on and drawing comparisons with what they hear from the other person. Consequently, joint interviews produce opportunities for a co-constructed account of the experience. The complexities of joint or individual interviewing in potentially sensitive topics has been described as contributing to a potentially perilous situation where consideration must be given to how researchers will manage their position 'in the middle' of two people in an intimate relationship (Forbat and Henderson, 2003). The stance adopted within this project, offering participants flexibility in their mode of interview, addresses this issue and left the decision in the hands of the participants.

Such methodological debates are central to the notion of relationality that we develop in this book. We consider the interview to be a site of the co-construction of experience where, between interviewer and interviewee(s), understandings are developed and created. The context of such discussions (including the presence and absence of other key people such as partners) will necessarily influence the accounts developed and the stories that can be told and those which remain silent. This connects with the constructionist approach adopted by family systems theorists, where meaning and language are recursively connected (Boston, 2000). Interviews are also considered the site of identity construction, where people negotiate and generate accounts of impact of cancer on their sense of self.

Excerpts from interview transcripts indicate whether the text is drawn from an individual or dyadic interview. This enables the reader to draw their own conclusions about the balance between public and private accounts being constructed at interview. Each extract also notes the type of cancer and which interview the quotation is taken from. This information is provided to help the reader contextualise the content of the discussion, related to the cancer diagnosis, and likely position of their experience in relation to diagnosis, treatment or follow-up care.

The interviews were designed to capture the range and depth of each person's experience. The interview guide was largely informed by four key policy themes (as described in Chapter 1), which were:

- people's experiences of involvement in their care (policy theme: patient involvement and self-care);

- care received within community and hospital-based settings and the impact of cancer on finances and employment (policy theme: shifting the balance of care);

- perceptions of care given by healthcare professionals (policy theme: culture of caring); and

- the involvement of family and friends (policy theme: role of carers/ partners).

Researchers asked open questions relating to each theme – for example, 'Can you tell me about your experiences of treatment?' – and encouraged the people affected by cancer to address the question in-depth by probing when appropriate.

Interviews lasted between 30 and 120 minutes. Interviews with people affected by cancer took place in the person's own home, although participants were also given the option of having the interview conducted at the University of Stirling or at the hospital where they were recruited.

Healthcare professional interviews

Following consent, healthcare professionals were interviewed by telephone in conjunction with the first interview with the person affected by cancer. These interviews focused on their perception of the experiences of the individual with cancer and the services provided. Twenty healthcare professionals consented to be interviewed. Interviews were conducted at a time that was convenient to them at either the point of diagnosis or treatment.

Data analysis

Initial analysis adopted a descriptive and thematic approach, which was theoretically informed by medical sociology and psychology and framed by recent health policy (see Chapter 1). There were five cyclical stages to analysis:

- each transcript read and re-read;
- themes and sub-themes relating to the key experience identified;
- data coded under each theme/sub-theme;
- coded data analysed;
- key concepts and issues identified.

During this iterative process, themes were expanded or collapsed into one another, sub-themes generated and data coded and re-coded. It was during this time, that key issues and concepts relating to the experience were identified. Finally, by comparing themes, issues and concepts across all key experiences, the researchers drew conceptual conclusions and made recommendations for cancer care policy, practice and further research. From this point an interpretative analysis, informed by systemic theory, was taken as a lens to the data, whereby the influences of context and relationships were considered as mediating and impacting upon people's accounts of cancer. The systemic theory was outlined in Chapter 1, with reference to family therapy as a distinct discipline that applies these notions in practice settings, to help elucidate accounts of their experience. Analytically, this approach shapes a relational gaze upon the data. In the following chapters, analysis moves between a broad approach to system theory (such as relationships with other patients in Chapter 5), to narrower approches drawing on sub-theories, which sit within a broader systemic approach. One example of this is in Chapter 8, where a specific theoretical approach of 'externalising' cancer is drawn upon to illustrate how people related to cancer.

Chapter 3

Interpersonal relationships: the family experience of cancer and its impact on family systems

This chapter examines the experience of cancer by centralising key interpersonal relationships, focusing on the family system. As described in the introduction, the focus on 'system' refers to the idea that individuals (and the problems they live with) cannot and should not be understood in isolation (Burnham, 1986). Fundamentally, there is a need to understand the entire context in which people experience and make sense of their illness, and particularly their interconnectedness and interrelationships with others. In the case of cancer, this means broadening out from a patient-centred approach to embracing the wider context in which the illness is experienced, including the relational aspects and impacts of cancer and cancer care across the family. Families, of course, vary in their structures and membership, and change across time and place; in this chapter 'family' is used to refer to those related through both biological and social ties.

For many years cancer research focused on the disease and biomedical approaches to drug treatments, with a growth in interest in the impact on the individual developing over the last thirty years. What remains notably absent from most of the literature is a considered approach to the individual with the illness in the context of their wider relationships. Some exceptions to this have voiced the need to identify the role of family relations, which has been picked up in cancer practice. As Sherman and Simonton (1999) indicate, we know that cancer occurs in a complex web of interpersonal relations, with implications and ramifications across family, friendship and work networks. As a marked move away from research that has focused on male partners of women with breast cancer (Vinkopur and Vinkopur-Kaplan, 1990), this chapter discusses a range of family relationships including parents, children and grandchildren.

Data from the interviews are used to develop two complementary theories: of the impact of cancer on relationship systems, and the impact of relational systems upon how cancer is experienced.

KEY ISSUES

- Families are one of the contexts in which cancer is experienced.
- Partners (spouses and life partners) played a number of key roles from pre-diagnosis onwards, for example, encouraging initial and subsequent appointments with the GP.
- Cancer affected relationships; and relationships affected the experience of cancer. In some families, cancer drew people together in a supportive web. In other families cancer was hidden to protect relatives.
- Some couples faced cancer together and developed a shared understanding of cancer care, which they reported had strengthened their relationship. Other couples reported the negative impact that cancer had on their intimate relationships.
- Despite an expressed need for support, some partners found it difficult to ask for help because they felt that they were meant to be strong for the person with cancer.
- Family members often lived at great distances from the person diagnosed with cancer, but were nevertheless affected by the disease.
- If services are to provide support for people with cancer, they can only do this by being mindful of the person's relational context. Supporting someone with cancer means supporting the family.

The role of family members

Family members were very clearly described as resources during times of illness. Many were felt to have an important and direct role in the experience of cancer, with relatives adapting their relating patterns to provide necessary support.

One participant's second utterance in the second interview starkly illustrates how important interpersonal relationships are viewed when cancer comes into someone's life:

> *Patient:* I have to say it was pretty tough indeed and thank God I had, I had [wife] eh, because I don't know how people would cope who didn't have a partner.
>
> *Partner:* He couldn't do anything for himself at that time. (38, colorectal cancer, interview 2, patient and partner)

At diagnosis

Partners and other family members play a number of roles starting often long before a cancer diagnosis was made, when symptoms were first noticed. Family members provided important initial encouragement to make appointments with the GP to investigate symptoms. Many partners encouraged both the recognition and investigation of symptoms before diagnosis:

> To be quite honest with you I would have rotted away and the inevitable would have happened to me … she pushed me and pushed me all the way and my daughter and my granddaughter, or I wouldn't be where I am today.
> (35, lung cancer, interview 1, patient and partner)

> I fought with him. I did everything. I was in tears and went myself and saw the doctor … an explosion. 'I'm not going, you hadn't any right discussing that.' So I said, 'If you'll not go for me what about your daughter? Your daughters and granddaughter?'(35, lung cancer, interview 1, partner only)

These quotations illustrate the role of the wider family network in facilitating initial presentation to the GP – involving both daughters and a granddaughter in expediting the eventual cancer diagnosis. Indeed, the partner above explicitly names family members in her speech as a rhetorical device to present a compelling case for Patient 35 to seek help. The centrality of close interpersonal relationships in health behaviours is clear to see.

Family members expressed just how aware they were of symptoms and worries, often for years, leading up to a diagnosis of cancer. The following extract is taken from an interview with a woman recently diagnosed with colorectal cancer and her daughter, following two years of symptoms:

> *Interviewer:* Would you tell me what the symptoms were?
> *Patient:* Oh, just waking up in the morning feeling like I had been hit with a sledge hammer, always got a sore stomach, my bowels and that were one minute constipated the next minute really loose. I'm just feeling really unwell. Tired, irritable as she'll tell you, didn't want to do nothing.
> *Interviewer:* Uh huh. For the past two years?
> *Patient:* Yes, it just got worse and worse and worse.
> *Interviewer:* And were you aware of your Mum's symptoms before the diagnosis?
> *Partner:* Uh huh, yeah we were. (06, colorectal cancer, interview 1, patient and daughter)

The daughter clearly indicates that the family had a good awareness of the impact of the symptoms. Indeed, the daughter even indicates that it is not just herself who has shared closely in these details, as her last utterance alerts the reader that others knew too: 'yeah *we* were'.

Despite encouraging the person with cancer to see a GP, this recognition of the potential salience of symptoms did not lessen the impact of the subsequent diagnosis on partners. Many patients and partners described feeling 'shocked', 'devastated' and 'distraught' on hearing the diagnosis. Some offered very powerful similes to describe their experience: 'It was like getting hit with a baseball bat' (02, colorectal cancer, interview 1, partner only). The daughter of one patient said 'I could describe the impact for me. I found it devastating. Erm really, really scary' (52, lung cancer, interview 1, patient and daughter). A partner expressed an immediate physical effect on them as they tried to process hearing the diagnosis: 'The two of us were shocked and I could actually, I thought I was going to faint because I could feel the blood draining out of me and everything was going wavy. And I thought, I can't even take in what he's saying' (17, colorectal cancer, interview 1, patient and partner).

Despite these very powerful reactions, family members nevertheless played an important role in supporting the person with the cancer at the point of diagnosis:

> It's good to have someone there to show you some support, em … you know there's, there's not a lot you can do when your, your, you're given a bombshell like that, I presume em … [pause], ah you know that, I'm a very guarded sort of individual, you know em, you don't, you don't like to feel exposed you don't like to feel vulnerable em, and I think quite often when you get hit with that sort of information em, you know you're sort of like, there should be questions that you're asking, and, and you don't ask, and maybe the person that's with you can sort of pick up on and make … maybe take the lead or, you know what I mean, just, just, just give you that bit of comfort sort of thing so, yeah, I think, I think what I do. (50, colorectal cancer, interview 2, patient only)

A partner, whose husband had recently been diagnosed with prostate cancer, reported that she had been told that there was unlikely to be anything significant wrong, and so was not present for the diagnosis. This led to some anxiety, since the information that he returned home with turned out to be confused. This partner identifies an important role in helping process information at times of stress:

> [The professionals said there would be] nothing untoward, made me think absolutely nothing wrong, that was a shock then! I would rather have worried. And I would've gone with him! […] And I would have thought more support to him. Because we actually got into a slight disagreement stage, because well he said 'oh I can't remember …' and I'm thinking, you…?! And then I felt sorry cos I thought he was in a bit of shock, cos you, you're told that when people are in shock when they're told they've got cancer. And although he seemed to come home with all the information, I don't think […] it's been shown to me that a couple of things got mixed up, confused, and that's caused us a bit of anxiety. (07, prostate cancer, interview 1, partner only)

Many partners identified themselves as primary information-givers, a role that appeared to be informally negotiated as a response to managing anxiety following the diagnosis. The following couple illustrate the reciprocal and complementary roles they have in managing new information:

> *Patient:* To be perfectly honest, we got booklets. You [talking to partner] read them, I just ignored them.
>
> *Partner:* I can understand. I read out bits to him, the really important bits. Basically I would say he doesn't want to read them.
>
> *Patient:* No, I don't want to know.
>
> *Partner:* You don't want to know, but I have learnt a lot reading the booklets. (01, colorectal cancer, interview 1, patient and partner)

Although there may be similarities in experience, such as being shocked, patient and partners responded differently to the diagnosis. Patients of course have a unique and well-defined role in terms of receiving medical interventions for the cancer. Partners, necessarily, have a different role that is often informally negotiated, in offering emotional, physical, practical and financial support. Many partners described the emotional support that they engaged in soon after diagnosis to help them influence, support and manage their feelings, as well as those of the person with the cancer diagnosis.

Families have histories that form a context for making sense of and responding to events in the present day, such as a cancer diagnosis. The following quotation shows how a father's death, over a decade ago, influenced one man's response to his sister's cancer diagnosis. The mother of the young woman who was diagnosed with cancer explains how her son reacted angrily:

> He sort of went a wee bit haywire that Friday night at youth club, he swore at some youngster and he said 'I know I lost it Mum when I said the word, the F word' and he said 'I just said to the other youth club worker I can't go further tonight I'm sorry I'll have to pack it in and go home, I can't go further tonight'. [He] went so very, very quiet, but it took back to him his Dad's death. He was about fourteen when his Dad died. (09, gynaecological cancer, interview 2, mother only)

The pressure of 'being there' and remaining 'positive' for the person with the cancer diagnosis was overwhelming at times: 'She's [daughter] trying to put on this brave face in front of me, but it fell down on Saturday night' (48, lung cancer, interview 1, patient only). Parallel to this, patients at times adopted a care-taker role of others. The following partner illustrates how his wife thinks of others:

> [She is] one of these people, someone'll phone up and say 'and how are you?', and she might have had the most bloody awful week and she'll say 'oh, I'm fine'. And I think no, you're not fine and that's your friend on the

phone, you know. How do you think your friend would feel if she thought that you weren't fine but you were saying it for her sake? (55, breast cancer, interview 2, patient and partner)

This quote illustrates the complexities of relationships when someone develops cancer. The patient is actively seen to manage the emotional well-being of others by presenting themselves as healthy and well to friends. Thus, although caregiving might traditionally be conceptualised as uni-directional from carer to patient, it is clear that the terrain is considerably more complex with people taking on a variety of roles in looking after each other's well-being.

During treatment

Many partners report increasing levels of strain as they progressed through the first year after diagnosis. One reason for this was because some partners had care responsibilities for older relatives, making cancer just one of a range of illnesses that were being managed within the family. With demographic analyses starkly indicating an ageing population, this is likely to become an increasingly familiar experience:

> I am actually beginning to really feel the strain ... I have my parents to look after, too, but now [Patient 01] is becoming more unwell I am finding it difficult ... I tried to explain to the receptionist at my father's surgery that I can't be there tomorrow, because I will be with [Patient 01] at [the hospital], but I also tried to let them know that I need help with my parents, because there is a lot to be done each day there. I am doing it, but it's getting too much because it's not simply cooking for them, it's cleaning, changing beds, shopping, filling in forms, getting their money for them ... (01, colorectal cancer, interview 1, patient and partner)

For some partners, the level of support they were providing to other family members resulted in compromising their own basic needs: 'it's being up and down and sleepless nights, and because I've been up with him or when he's sleeping, sometimes I can't sleep, I'm just up to maybe three, four ... I'm tired, I just want to spend maybe perhaps the whole day in bed, you know?' (39, colorectal cancer, interview 2, patient and partner).

A range of family supports were named as available during treatment, and were framed as helpful and appropriate. Managing this provision (and acceptance) of support required the use of some deft footwork. Patients effectively managed family members' identities by suggesting that help post-diagnosis is consistent with the support they were given pre-diagnosis. People affected by cancer therefore had a role in constructing delicate accounts of the impact of cancer on family members' behaviour.

The following quotation illustrates how people with cancer managed the construction of their relationship when talking about how family members have supported them through treatment:

> I do get more breathless now, em, I don't walk the same distances as what I would have walked, em, it, I, I think I do tire a bit easier, em, but it certainly hasn't changed, we haven't let it change too much in the family, if I'm tired I'll just say 'look I'm tired, I need a nap,' then [my husband will] take the children, but he did that before anyway ... so I, I wouldn't have said there's been that much change with the way we deal with the children, em, [my husband's] mum tends to take the children a little bit more em, to give me a break and my sister has taken them to sort of like let me have a sleep when I was getting tired. (50, colorectal cancer, interview 2, patient only)

This speaker works hard to present an acceptable account of how her illness is managed within the family. She manoeuvres between describing minimal changes in the family, to stating how her husband helps out. This is then shored up with identity work for the husband, as she expresses that his support is not unusual. The changes in how family members support her are described primarily as involving the extended family, including her mother-in-law and sister. Overall, it is clear that cancer has impacted upon how family members assist each other, and how a change in one part of the family has led to changes throughout the family system.

Beyond Treatment

The role of family members changed as the patient progressed from diagnosis, through treatment and then into follow-up care; adapting to acute and chronic phases of the disease and its subsequent impact on the patient. The importance of reciprocity among family and friends was particularly palpable during the post-treatment phase. Through the course of the final interview, many partners found that even after treatment had finished, the emotional and physical toll continued. Several people reported that fear and anxiety could 'come rushing back', particularly when the patient began to get symptoms from everyday illnesses, such as colds. Other participants spoke of continuing difficulties balancing family life, work, relationships, commitments and responsibilities. The following speaker highlights a number of issues central to many people's accounts regarding continued anxiety. It is significant that the speaker is the partner of a woman with breast cancer, and is so clearly articulating the ongoing impacts on both of them over the longer term:

> There's a feeling that it's okay. Treatment's finished, right, bye, see you. Well no. See you for the next 5 years or whatever, every so often, but it's kind of like the process is through, so jump off the conveyor belt and go

about your business as it were … so we need to kind of get a bit proactive and make sure that … we get a bit of direction and a bit of, I wouldn't say reassurance, but just basically how the process is going and what the next stages are, because you know, ok we've finished all the treatment but … is it still there? Is it not there? Can it come back? Can it not come back? What happens when we've finished this course of treatment, if there's no more, well, what do we do? … it's a period of uncertainty just now … we've gone through it all but you know, what's next? (12, breast cancer, interview 3, patient and partner)

For many couples, cancer remained a central organising component of life after treatment. Uncertainty and fear of recurrence were critical concerns for both patient and partner, underlined in the following partner account: 'In the heavy moments and the moments when we're tired I don't say it and neither does she, but we have said it to one another once or twice, just wonders where is it going to pop up next?' (09, gynaecological cancer, interview 3, patient and partner). The notion of tiredness is recruited into this account, indicating the need for emotional strength to face these challenges together. The statement reinforces the idea that cancer is jointly owned and experienced, as they hold together in their reticence to speak of their worries.

Partners expressed difficulty moving on from the experience of cancer:

I'm actually finding it harder as time goes on, believe it or not. I find my life's changed completely, it's not his fault, don't get me wrong, I mean I love [partner], I'll always be here for him, always look after him, but I've got my bad days as well. You know some days I feel I need to get away from here for a wee while, but don't get me wrong, it doesn't stop me going out at all. But when I go out I feel guilty. I can't really relax. (63, lung cancer, interview 3, patient and partner)

This passage illustrates the powerful impact of cancer over the longer term. Despite treatment being over, things are 'harder as times goes on'. The speaker appears conflicted, expressing their love for their partner, yet guilt at going out and getting on with life. Additionally, this passage highlights that a year on from the cancer diagnosis, relaxation was not forthcoming, indicating the powerful long-term effects on relatives, not just the person with the diagnosis.

A number of people affected by cancer expressed a need for support, but found difficulty asking for it. The following speaker identifies cultural and gender issues with asking for help (Scottishness and masculinity), but recognises that they weren't supported as fully as he would have liked by his family:

Partner: You kind of hope that people would be perceptive enough to say 'I wonder how [he is] feeling' and 'give him a ring and see if he wants to get together'. You don't like to phone up and ask and reveal that you're needy in any way ... maybe a man thing, maybe a Scottish thing ... because you're not asking for help people maybe assume that you might be alright, and it would have been nice to have a bit more contact ... I don't think I would have liked support from people I didn't know

Interviewer: No, but in terms of family and ...

Partner: Yeah. (55, breast cancer, interview 3, partner only)

Looking back at the past year's experiences, this speaker clearly identifies a strong desire for more support (from unidentified friends/family), which had not been forthcoming.

The presence of the possibility of death led to participants making preparations for their family. Practical tasks such as making a will and arranging bank accounts were described in relational terms:

Interviewer: So, being given that information, have you done, have you talked to anybody about dying, about bereavement?

Patient: I've talked to my wife.

Interviewer: Yeah, and what, what have you talked to her about?

Patient: Well just to, try and get my bank accounts in order and things like that. We'd normally have different, different bank accounts, we're going through the process of getting it all in joint account. Just for it'll be helpful for, for her like. (68, lung cancer, interview 1, patient only)

Managing the intricacies of discussing death within families is a delicate process. As well as the practicalities, there are more ephemeral issues that families contend with including existential conversations. The following speaker suggests that she is being realistic when talking about her own death, whereas her mother refers to this as being pessimistic:

I've been really realistic, my mum, she thinks I'm being pessimistic because she, I keep talking about dying and things like, and she's like 'would you stop talking', and I was like 'I know but that's not, that's being optimistic as well, because I need to know, I need to', 'cause I went away on Friday to do my will and I'm going back to get it signed on Wednesday, and I go for surgery on Thursday and my mum's like, 'oh wills' and stuff and I says 'I know but, I might die', 'you don't know that', and I says 'I need to, to do these things for me, I need to get them sorted out, you know and I've got like this massive pile of paperwork that I've got things to fill in and send off and that I've got to do that I haven't, I've been putting off, putting off, putting off and I really need to do them, so, it's just things like that' and, and I think that's not how she dealt with it, although we did have, her and I did have some more kind of deep and meaningful discussions about death and dying than she had with the rest of the family em, but I think and, but I don't think she likes to hear me talking about it. (70, breast cancer, interview 1, patient only)

Each of the excerpts above reinforce a clear message articulated by patients and family members in this study: the impact of cancer reverberates across whole families, rather than solely for the individual with the diagnosis. People's family relationships provide a context in which cancer is experienced and understood. In the following section, the further impact of cancer on changing relationships is discussed.

Changing relationships

Cancer takes its toll on interpersonal relationships. Many respondents spoke of how cancer had impacted upon them and changed their relationships with people close to them. As Rolland surmises 'a serious health crisis can awaken family members to opportunities for more satisfying, fulfilling relationships with each other' (1994: 10). A systemic understanding of illness suggests that cancer may precipitate centripetal and centrifugal forces. Centripetal forces draw family members in toward each other, and may occur at the onset of illness or during an acute phase; centrifugal forces by contrast are those which create distance between family members, which may occur during chronic phases of the condition. One partner reported how cancer had created a barrier to open communication between himself and his partner:

> *Partner:* Every time I found myself feeling a certain way, the last thing I felt I wanted to do was to put any pressure on [my partner] at all because relative to what [my partner] was going through, anything I was going through was child's play
>
> *Interviewer:* Like you say, you were the healthy one
>
> *Partner:* That's right, so I think it was a strange thing to have to do, to not say what was on your mind, to keep any worries to yourself but it was the right thing to do and it wasn't too difficult for me to do that I mean I had to keep reminding myself [my partner] is going through this cancer treatment, I haven't got cancer so you know anything that I'm concerned about pales into insignificance but it was a strange thing to have to do because good relationships are all about saying what's on your mind … so maybe that was wrong of me to do that because she did say to me at the beginning of the whole process 'you know I want you to talk to me if you've got anything on your mind' and I thought about it a few times and I thought, no you've got enough to think about yourself, you know I'll just keep that to me and I won't add to your worries. (55, breast cancer, interview 2, partner only)

For the same couple, questions were raised about how attractive the woman remained to her partner, following treatment:

The only thing that he, the Freudian thing he said which I shouldn't really say it but I suppose it obviously em, hurt me was, he has this habit of, of showing my photo to everybody, anybody he meets 'oh this is the, you know the beautiful woman I live with', and he was at em, doing his job and showing my photo again to a work colleague or something and he, he was telling me 'and I was showing this photo of you in, showing this photo to people to show how beautiful you were'; this was after I lost my hair and I, I said 'how do mean how beautiful I *was*' ... I mean 'cause I never think I'm beautiful anyway but you know he always has and he, you know you could just see h–, as he said it, you could see him take a big breath in thinking 'oh my God, I've ... will she notice what I've just said?' ... and I'm laughing about it now, but it, you know it really hurt me at the time and I've forgiven him for it 'cause he's wonderful but I haven't forgotten it. (55, breast cancer, interview 2, patient only)

For some couples, the cancer meant that their social lives became more aligned. The speaker below indicates that he found that nightclubs were no longer appropriate for him, while he managed the side-effects of treatment and he spent more time with his partner engaging in social events which she enjoys:

> *Patient:* One thing I did find as well is that, before we were pretty sociable, we were out night-clubbing and we were out with our friends and stuff like that, eh, since I've become, became ill, we've done a lot more things, we're self together, like that, I probably wouldn't have been in a rush to, like going to the theatre, I mean, I didn't mind going to the theatre for some things, but I mean, I found myself going in to see shows with [partner], 'cause she likes the theatre.
>
> *Partner:* So he's coming along with me now! [laughs] ... He would never have dreamt of going before.
>
> *Patient:* But I was, it was an alternative to going to the nightclub and standing up, you can go to the theatre you could sit down. (28, colorectal cancer, interview 2, patient and partner)

For one participant, the cancer had impacted upon her relationship with her teenage son. At a time of transition for her child, managing her ill health had led to a questioning process for him. The following extract illustrates how her son was 'lugging' (listening) in to conversations in an attempt to learn more about his mother's illness:

> *Patient:* I never thought he was listening, he's thirteen, I should have known he'd been lugging in somewhere, he says 'does that mean you're not going to be here for my eighteenth birthday'. I says 'don't be stupid, you picked it up wrong', I says 'yes that's just one doctor said that', I said

'I'll be here for your eighteenth birthday', I says 'that's just one stupid doctor'. I says 'my doctor doesn't say that', I try to keep that from them, he's too young to understand what we're talking about but he actually he'd been lugging in.

Partner: He's a sensitive lad as well.

Patient: And I said I'd be here for his eighteenth so I've got to stay another five years. (06, colorectal cancer, interview 3, patient and partner)

Thus at a time when many teenagers are beginning the process of individuation and autonomy from families, cancer can provoke a shift toward less separation and dependence, illustrating the centripetal forces at play.

For some couples, their intimate relationships had changed as a consequence of both emotional and physical elements of the disease and treatments. Cancer had obstructed some couples' sex life; for example, treatment side-effects for some men with prostate cancer had led to impotence. Some couples discussed this together with the interviewer, whereas others used individual interviews as an opportunity to talk about intimacy. The following quotation illustrates one partner's lament at the impact treatment has had on their sexual relationship:

It's been a little issue for me and he wouldn't want to talk about it so I sort of bring it up and then obviously the urinary leakage that's something he deals with and I admire him and he knows that because I suffer from some stress bladder incontinence, so its quite funny 'cos we can sort of laugh about that but on the sexual side, I feel that wasn't something that I was prepared enough for to be honest and wanting to be positive for him because your bottom line is you want the cancer out and you want the person to have a long life and therefore you're prepared that they may have to be changes and it almost seems like it would be petty of me to, but then you have to be truthful to yourself and say its not like we don't have a sex life now but I think its more of a thing for me because he's been through the surgery and he's glad to have come through it and he's fully occupied at work. (07, prostate cancer, interview 3, partner only)

For many people in this study then, cancer had changed their relationships with family members and heightened focus on specific elements of their relationships. Many people, particularly couples, reported that a significant shift had occurred for them in facing cancer together.

Facing cancer together

The previous section explored how cancer impacted upon relationships. This section suggests that relationships can affect the experience of cancer; indeed, relationships are one of the contexts in which cancer is negotiated. A common feature in interviews was the construction of cancer as something that is managed together, particularly for partners/spouses. This joint ownership of cancer again centralises the importance of understanding cancer in a wide relational context, as people position themselves to be more or less involved in its meaning and implications for their lives (Illingworth *et al.*, 2009).

Many partners actively and keenly constructed a shared understanding of their experience of cancer. This was often made clear by people's use of the pronoun 'we' as they described managing the consequences of cancer (emphasis added in the following): 'I think *we* have been able to manage a routine, I think *we* have been able to keep positive attitude, I think *we* have played it probably right with the kids … *we* have now got to the stage where *we*'re kind of trying to put ourselves, you know, first, as much as possible …' (12, breast cancer, interview 1, partner only). The mother of one patient expressed a similar idea, constructing cancer as an enemy that is out to 'get her daughter'. She articulates an idea of a joint fight against cancer:

> When she [the daughter diagnosed with cancer] came in on the Friday I just grabbed her in my arms when she collapsed in the doorway and I thought, 'no, no, you're not getting my daughter, no,' and I think I must have been screaming out 'no' and I thought 'come on, come on I've got to pull myself together she needs support, we're fighting this.' (09, gynaecological cancer, interview 2, mother only)

Such talk begins to construct cancer as something which is jointly owned and experienced. This was visible for some participants as they reframed their focus on getting through treatment together and agreement that the future holds more than cancer for them:

> We don't know what's coming … everything else has been kind of a sideshow and of lesser importance, so to be honest that's not the thing we are focusing on, we knew … she got out the operation really well so that's great, but it's now moved on … I think if this, if this was the be all and end all, if this was it, then we would probably have a lot more to say, and a lot more to talk about, but because we know there's far greater challenges ahead, it's like ok, we've done it, move on, good … (12, breast cancer, interview 2, partner only)

A further patient illustrated the extent to which cancer had impacted upon his family and friendship networks:

> A lot of people say, 'you're going through this hard time', but the thing that they don't realise is, it's not just me it's everybody … you'll have heard in the discussions with other people, that … the family, I mean [my partner's] been a rock through the whole thing … my mum, my dad, eh, [partner's]

mum and dad, my brother and sisters, and the family and the friends as well, I mean, I've got, we've got good friends and they would be on the phone at least once a week just checking to see how you were, and, they're all getting a bit of stress as well, I mean they're all concerned about you ... but you've got your friends that are like, well, so, and I mean, everybody's going through it, I mean they've been really concerned about her and eh, I tell them to take her on holidays and stuff like that. (28, colorectal cancer, interview 2, patient and partner)

It is possible to see in this passage further articulation of the joint ownership of the disease, and impact upon partners. The final utterance marks out what can be interpreted as a stance that the partner is in need of a holiday (used as a synonym or proxy for break/respite) because of the impact of cancer on her. The patient's encouragement that holidays are taken can equally be seen as part of an ongoing reciprocity within the relationship where they both take care of each other.

The notion of togetherness through cancer was apparent in some accounts, as people spoke about the mutual support that the patient and partner provided for each other. For such couples, the shared experience of cancer enhanced and consolidated their relationship: 'We really, em, we actually feed off each other, eh, under these darkest of circumstances in a really positive way em, I mean we laugh a lot, and there are tears, but there's a whole lot more laughter than, than, than there is em, tears ...' (69, lung cancer, interview 2, patient and partner).

At other times, the relationship was used as a vehicle for managing difficulties (as well as a site for those difficulties). For example, the patient in one couple worked to negatively shape his interaction with his partner in the hope that this would lessen her emotional difficulties should his prognosis be poor:

> *Patient:* In my mind if I fall out with her, I just get crabby to her all the time, if anything happens to me, it'll ease the burden.
> *Partner:* That's his attitude to me was, 'I want you to fall out, just fall out with me, don't talk to me much, I can't handle that', I says 'that'll not make any difference to me, I'll still be here.' 'But I don't want you to talk to me, fall out with me.' I mean, that's quite hard to handle, you know, when he's argumentative, just doesn't want me. (63, lung cancer, interview 1, patient and partner)

In this way, the relationship is moulded to perform functions for those involved. In the above case it is used strategically to try and shift them out of a contented position into a less satisfactory one, where (if the patient were to die) there would be less for the partner to grieve for. Facing cancer together was therefore something which led to a mindful manipulation of their relationship and an attempt to precipitate the centrifugal forces that would distance the partner. The conscious articulation of this process indicates how centrally the patient places the relationship, and the patient's wish to ease the emotional toll for her.

One partner described the process of taking on the positive attitude that their husband had adopted and how this impacted upon her relationship with cancer and him: 'The first day the doctor said to him it's a tumour and I was like ooof. We came out and he [husband] says "how are you feeling?" How are you feeling? He said "I'm absolutely fine". [...] So that day when we came out he said "I'm absolutely fine". I said "right. I'm fine"'(35, lung cancer, interview 1, patient and partner). Thus, there was a process of negotiating how they would relate to the cancer, and the uptake of a positive attitude; if the patient had decided to be positive, this was a stance that the partner must also therefore take. This symbiotic response underscores the importance of identifying cancer as affecting whole family systems, rather than identifying it as a disease which affects just the individual with the cancer.

Professionals also offered their views on family relationships, reflecting what they had noticed in how couples relate with each other:

> He deals with things by being a bit flippant. His wife was a bit more shocked, or she appeared more shocked. And she didn't cry, but she was a bit, filled up a wee bit ... the wife ... reacted probably the way we would expect people to react to news like that. More than he did. I think she will calm him down. I think she'll see that as being her role. And being the person that's there to give him a little support and I don't know if that's the way it's been all along in their relationship ... she'll neglect herself a bit. I feel I probably need to support her more. (17, colorectal cancer, clinical nurse specialist)

This nurse specialist constructs a clear role too for the patient's wife as calming him and providing support. The professional also demonstrates recognition that her own role is much wider than supporting the individual with the diagnosis, and that at times, her main focus may be more appropriately directed toward family members.

The familial experience of cancer is underlined strongly by the daughter of one patient, as the disease is located within the wider family context and time of year:

> *Daughter:* We knew something was wrong with Mum and I kind of had it in the back of my head, but I didn't really, you know, think about it if you like. But the day that she was diagnosed we just buried my husband's sister-in-law who had died of cancer, and one of our friends is in the hospital at the moment with cancer and eh, well they are going back in February as well so, it was just sort of, you know, well we just picked Mum up after the funeral but we tried not to dwell on it too much. Because Mum said she wasn't going to tell anyone over Christmas and New Year but she did, she told everyone.

> *Patient:* If I had kept it from them over Christmas and New Year the four
> of them, they wouldn't have thanked me. They would have gone hell for
> leather, 'why didn't you tell us, why did you keep it to yourself' and that's
> the reason why I decided to. (06, colorectal cancer, interview 1, patient and daughter)

This illustrates the interconnections of family members, and the lived experience
of cancer as one that is shared within a family, rather than the business of just one
individual. Despite, or perhaps because of, the time of year, consideration was given to
how the diagnosis may impact upon others. This passage also illustrates the negotia-
tions around how and when concerns are faced together, or alone (which is explored
in the next section).

Some participants wished to explicitly describe the positive impact that cancer
had had on their family relationships and friendships:

> I think it's brought us closer together [...] I've got my sister over here and
> my mother in Skye ... I don't think we've ever been as close and I know
> from my sister and I's point of view it's, it's one of the great things that's
> come out of it because we do get closer and closer, and she's just been so
> wonderfully supportive and em, and my mother too I mean she always
> is, always has been and, you know she's, she's always great, and friends as
> well, em, I've seen more of everybody since this. (55, breast cancer, interview 2,
> patient only)

This notion of bringing families together was a strong theme. However, not all experiences of cancer were felt to be both positive and shared. Some people felt as though
they were very much facing cancer alone.

Facing cancer alone

A balance between facing cancer together and facing it alone is managed by people
who struggle with well-documented concerns (Brechin *et al.*, 1998) about becoming dependent upon others. For some, the diagnosis had precipitated a desire to
distance themselves from others: 'I really don't want people to be doing things for
me, I'd like to do as many thing for myself for as long as I possibly can!' (43, prostate
cancer, interview 2, patient and partner). The desire for some individuals to face cancer alone
was overwhelming. Many participants indicated that they did not want to burden
others with knowledge of the diagnosis. For the following speaker, in addition to
not telling his golfing friends of his illness, he had also protected his daughter from
knowing of his cancer:

> *Partner:* You haven't told your golf cronies have you?
> *Patient:* They're not, well they've been in, the know, [...] I said 'I have to go
> I've got an appointment' but they don't know the extent. I mean there's
> no, eh. My family don't, I mean my daughter doesn't know. She's, well

there's no point in, until we know what's the prognosis is and so on and whether they're going to zap me or, eh, give me hormone. (64, prostate cancer, interview 1, patient and partner)

This protectionism was common, and the impact of cancer on family communication was clear across many of the interviews. Patients often had a limited number of people with whom they would speak openly to about the cancer, and frequently had specific relatives who they did not wish to disclose their diagnosis to. The following lengthy quote illustrates how powerful this is for people diagnosed with cancer, in the context of family relationships:

> *Interviewer:* You said lots of people tell you to tell your daughter. Who are these people, is that family or healthcare professionals?
>
> *Patient:* My family, my friends. It's, 'have you still not told [my daughter], have you still not told [my daughter]'. I'm like that look this is my choice, if anybody knows [my daughter]. I know my daughter, I know how it will affect her, I know what will happen and she would just go right into a blue thunk. 'My Daddy, my Daddy, my Daddy, my Daddy', and I don't want that. I mean, what is the old saying, no news is what?
>
> *Interviewer:* Good news.
>
> *Patient:* Yes. Then why not leave her, ignorance is bliss. To use two. But there's no way, I didn't bring her into the world to make her unhappy, so there is no way I am going to give her news. As I say.
>
> *Interviewer:* So you are protecting her in a way?
>
> *Patient:* I mean I've always done that anyway. That's what I am there for. I mean if your father can't protect you there's not much bloody point being here is there, you're just a waif, you're just an orphan, you're just a child that's lost. I've always been there when she needed me. Both of them, but to me, there's no way. My Granny used to have an old saying 'if I can't bring a smile to your face, I'll never bring a tear to your eye'. Right. And I feel that. Who wants a Daddy coming up and saying 'wait until I tell you this, oh no I'm ill, oh I'm ill, don't think you will be seeing your Da for a long time'. You know what I mean that's ludicrous; she isn't here for that purpose. She's here to enjoy herself, you know what I mean. And if she thinks her Daddy's well and, I'm happy with that. (36, lung cancer, interview 2, patient and partner)

For the above speaker then, his position as a father and associated scripts regarding his responsibility for protecting his daughter was dominant in his experience of facing cancer alone.

For other patients, a construction of feeling alone was challenged by family members. The following speaker presents herself as 'coping' which is defined, albeit reluctantly, as not crying in front of people. The granddaughter challenges this isolationist view of the patient's disease, expressing that she had borne witness to her grandmother's crying, indicating that she is not alone with her sadness:

> *Patient:* I'm finding it hard to deal with at the moment. I mean I hadn't … I think I'm coping quite well you know … as I say it's not as if I've never had surgery or anything like that but … [tone of voice is very sad]
>
> *Granddaughter:* Nan, you've done nothing but cry for two weeks, be honest …
>
> *Patient:* Well of and on, you know I haven't cried in front of people, y'know I mean it's …'
>
> *Granddaughter:* Am I not … am I nobody like … you cry in front of me all the time Nan. (13, colorectal cancer, interview 1, patient and granddaughter)

Other patients felt that the onset of cancer and treatment had led to rejection by their partner, so facing cancer alone was not chosen by the patient. One woman felt very unsupported by her husband after her breast cancer diagnosis. Though she was not literally abandoned, she felt as though he was emotionally and practically unavailable for her:

> To be quite honest I've felt very abandoned by my husband and that has come to a head em, at, I'm still looking for my cuddle when I was diagnosed. […] we've no sexual problems, we don't, because we don't have any sex, he won't touch me. When the first time he heard that I'd got a lump, he turned his back on me, and I think it's still turned. He's better to me now than what I was going through chemo, 'cause he can see this tiredness, fatigue come over, he's not too bad most of the time. When I was going through chemo he was waiting on me getting ill before he helped, even though I was retching and being sick, I was still expected to cook tea and do everything, he's a lot better than that, but em, mostly reassuring, forget it, you know. So I've, I think that's caused a lot of sadness that I have felt very alone and abandoned you know, I know my daughter tries to help, she does, but she's got four children, you cannot dump too much on her. I live with this man, he knows I'm sad, he knows I'm upset. He says I'm 'wallowing', I probably am. (21, breast cancer, interview 3, patient only)

For this individual then, the experience of cancer was one that had clearly impacted on her relationship with her husband. This is defined as taking place prior to diagnosis, with the detection of the lump marking the end of physical and sexual contact between them. Her sense of isolation is broader than sexual intimacy though, as she sees scope for her daughter to fill some of the space and provide her with reassurance. In the final utterance, she also marks out the difference in how she relates to her illness and how her husband does, expressed by the notion of 'wallowing' in the illness, and its role perhaps as a defining characteristic.

Other family members took their cues from the individual with cancer. The relational meaning of cancer is underlined by a healthcare professional who articulates the importance of understanding how cancer is experienced within the family.

> Her family, her son was very positive ... she lives alone. He did visit frequently but she was a very independent lady ... she didn't sit back and become a cancer patient ... she wanted to carry on and keep life as normal as possible. Baked oatcakes, I always remember every time she came in she said oh she was well enough to bake oatcakes so that kept everybody happy ... and that seemed to be the yard mark for the family – if she still managed to carry on while doing these tasks they were delighted. (20, gynaecological cancer, clinical nurse specialist)

The wider family

Interviews within this study were limited to people with cancer and their nominated other, who was often a partner/spouse. Members of wider circles of family or friendship networks were not purposively sampled for interview. However, despite this, the significance of the cancer experience for the wider family was a recurrent feature through the interviews. Although there were many dimensions to the response of the wider family to the cancer experience, it was clear that patient experiences of cancer and cancer care could not be isolated from either personal or wider family relationships.

One woman spoke of her anguish at telling her children about having cancer investigations and a potentially poor prognosis, a feature echoed widely across the cohort of participants: 'I'm sat here thinking, oh I'm going to go and I going to have to tell the children what, and what if it is something and it, and it probably isn't but then what if I'm not here next year, you know what I mean and what ...' (70, breast cancer, interview 2, patient only). Another woman makes a connection to how she managed when her own mother became ill, and reflects on how her children are coping with her own cancer. She clearly indicates concern about how her cancer is putting undue stress on her children (bairns):

> Now I mean my daughter she can't sleep at night 'cause she's so worried about me and the boys, they are only babies, it was a shame like, and my wee boy is away, the bairns aren't coping, and that's what gets me so upset 'cause I can cope, I can, but when I see it in them it's like, it's terrible, but I can't remember me being like that fifteen years ago with my mum ... I just feel as though my illness is putting stress on my bairns and I don't like that, I can cope with me having cancer, but I can't cope with my bairns ... having to watch me go though what I'm going through, I don't know what they're going through. (26, gynaecological cancer, interview 1, patient only)

Later on in the interview she indicates that her responsibility seems even more pressing, since the children have no contact with their father, making her the only parent figure they have to rely upon. The meaning of cancer is thereby mediated by relationships that are absent as well as those that are present:

> *Patient:* What's going to happen to them, what kind of state, emotional, their head, what's their head going to be like, their childhood and then this and I'm no going to be here, no that am, am I going to be here? But just in case, that's why I worry about them so much, if ah wasn't but am ah, know what I mean?
>
> *Interviewer:* Have they got good contact with their dads?
>
> *Patient:* No, it's just me
>
> *Interviewer:* So, it's just you, so you really feel like the responsibility of, yeah ...
>
> *Patient:* And it's shite me putting that responsibility onto their wee shoulders it's, a vicious bloody circle, they would do alright you know, it's not as they were, aw it's a bloody shame [...], there's hundreds of families out there like that, you know we're doing alright, we just get on with it, at the end oh the day it's their fathers' faults for no being there. (26, gynaecological cancer, interview one, patient only)

For this speaker then, the family's life-cycle position is critical in mediating the meaning of illness. Cancer has occurred at a time in her life when her major role and responsibility is around parenting, with cancer creating a disruption to this key task. Another participant having treatment for breast cancer spoke of its impact on her ability to have more children:

> *Patient:* I'm not allowed to have children for five years 'cause I'm taking this tablet and I mean, I might not have wanted to have [more] children anyway, but I'm not allowed ...
>
> *Interviewer:* But you might have.
>
> *Patient:* You know what I mean, so it's, it's, just ...
>
> *Interviewer:* Taking choices away and, and changing your ...
>
> *Patient:* Uh huh, and I know that some people like have, like due to this they have to lose their ovaries and stuff and I mean a lot of people who, I mean I'm quite lucky because I've got children, a lot of people like, because they delay their family, you know they've not got children you know and it's, it's ... or some people find out when they're pregnant and things like that you know, but, so in that sense I'm lucky, but it's just that, I might have wanted to make that choice and, and I'm not getting to now, you know. Well not for the next five years, and even then, I don't know in five years time, I mean it can put you into, through the menopause,

so I might, that might be it, I might never get a chance to have [more] children. (70, breast cancer, interview 2, patient only)

Thus the wider family can be thought of not solely as those members who are related through blood or marriage, but also an imagined or hoped-for future family, including children and (as other speakers suggested) partners.

One of the consequences of viewing the impact of cancer as wider than purely the individual with the disease is an awareness of how the patient copes with more than their own feelings about cancer. In this case, family dynamics impact on the individual with cancer and change the way they relate to and report their symptoms to others. Many people with cancer often discussed the wider family's ability to cope with the illness:

If I'm feeling like 'cack', I would tend not to really say … 'I've got a sore head today' … basically you don't want them worrying, you know what I mean? (50, colorectal cancer, interview 2, patient only)

My daughter … she can't sleep at night because she's so worried … the kids aren't coping and that's what gets me so upset, 'cause I can cope, I can, but when I see it in them it's like, it's terrible … I'm coping with it alright, it's like, I feel as though my family aren't … and that upsets me, if I can cope with it how the hell can they not? It's a vicious bloody circle. (26, gynaecological cancer, interview 2, patient only)

This woman's account troubles the straightforward notion of a joint ownership/ experience of the disease. Here, she positions family members as taking on *too much* of the impact of the disease, such that their emotional reactions are more extreme than her own. The notion of the 'vicious circle' builds up a picture of increasing angst among the family where their responses and reactions create a further context of distress. Thus, we see a recursive feedback loop of difficulty within some families, as they strive to make sense of and respond to the cancer which subsequently creates new levels of meaning for other members of the family.

The impact of cancer was associated with a range of feelings, including guilt: '… they've got to cramp their style because of me …' (44, lung cancer, interview 2, patient and partner). Other people spoke of their strategies to minimise the impact of cancer. One participant spoke of their perception of how their son had managed to limit the impact of cancer on him: 'My oldest son … I think he's just keeping a wide berth …' (08, breast cancer, interview 2, patient only).

Some other people with cancer described the wider family as a positive source of support and encouragement, and often preferred this over formal support services. Others, such as the following patient, were more ambivalent about family support: 'They have rallied round me and given me a lot of, given me support, but we don't go into depth about, about "the big C", 'cause I would get up and walk away' (46, lung cancer, interview 2, patient).

Several interviewees spoke of how cancer has drawn the family closer together.

> *Patient:* The one thing I will say, is it's brought my family closer together. There is more interaction between them.
>
> *Interviewer:* All right, good.
>
> *Patient:* My brother phones my sister, my sister phones my other brother.
>
> *Interviewer:* About you, or?
>
> *Patient:* About me, right. Honestly, I didn't mean to be, you know what I mean, Superstar. No, there's a kind of much more openness between them now. (36, lung cancer, interview 2, patient only)

This same speaker appears earlier in the chapter, also illustrating how he had been reluctant to tell his daughter of his cancer diagnosis. The complex contradictions of living with cancer in a family context are thus brought to light as he celebrates the closeness that his illness has brought, while lamenting the stress this could place on his daughter if she were to learn of his cancer.

The global impact of cancer on families

A large number of participants spoke of the geographical distances their families live across. This diasporic relational element appeared to make a difference to how cancer was experienced. Many of the participants had close family (such as siblings or adult children) living at considerable distances, including across the breadth of the British Isles, America and Australia. Managing these distances became a mediating factor in how and whether family members were informed of the cancer, and subsequently in relatives' abilities to offer support and integrate this role into their own lives. Geography and distance thereby influence the process of negotiating a familial response to cancer.

> *Interviewer:* In terms of your family and friends, what impact do you think it's had on, on them?
>
> *Patient:* [My niece] in Colorado, God bless her, [she] is a 'need to know' type, she's only ten years younger than I, she's a need to know type and her daughter and her son-in-law are both nurses, so what I didn't tell my niece, she would have ferreted it out of her family, so my reflexologist has been told absolutely everything; she was the only person who was ever told everything. The eh, nobody else was told, although they suspected, they were not given the definite news until I knew what the definite news was, no I mean she said, 'oh if your having an op, I'm coming over', you know, and it's almost impossible in her high-powered job, you know, and I thought oh God bless her. We're her only family now, her mother died at Christmas, so it's really only my sister and my niece, who's more like a sister who are actually em, 'in it', as it were.

Partner: Aye, but the other relations, I mean eh, they're obviously interested.
(31, gynaecological cancer, interview 2, patient and partner)

Another couple reflect on how difficult a parent's cancer diagnosis is for their adult daughter, who lives in England:

Partner: Our daughter is very, em, her being a nurse I suppose, and she actually, she used to do one-to-one paediatric nursing with children that had terminal cancer so but it got too much for her eventually, you know, she says it was difficult to leave it and not bring it home. So now she's a school nurse but she is very supportive, the only problem both for her and for us is she lives in England, which makes it difficult. I think her father sometimes finds her a bit overpowering but as I've said to him you've got to remember she is, you know.

Patient: The mileage in-between us.

Partner: She feels, I'm sure she feels isolation which is another thing that I'm sure something you should talk about for the family that live away it is difficult. (46, lung cancer, interview 1, patient and partner)

Telephone contacts play a critical role in enabling people affected by cancer to keep in touch with family located across the UK, and all round the world:

They've all been very concerned, well my brother he's been up visiting me and I just had my brother from England up. My sister in England she was continually phoning when I was in hospital and I've got a sister in Australia and she's been phoning a few times. They all feel so helpless and the vast majority are not even in the area so there's, they just phone and I've been phoning my sister a few times in England and kind of crying, or swearing down the phone to her, so that's what's helped with the emotions as well because I said to her a few times 'look I'm sorry about this', she said 'look that's what we're here for', she said 'we can't do anything for you physically we're here for you on the phone' and same as my big sister abroad and my brother in England have been crying sometimes and swearing the next time and they've been there for me boosting me up. (09, gynaecological cancer, interview 2, patient only)

For some participants, health professionals were aware of the distances between patients and families, and about how individuals managed diagnostic disclosure. One GP indicates how one patient was unaware of her sister's cervical cancer, until her own diagnosis.

Actually interestingly enough her sister in Australia had, had a hysterectomy for cancer of the cervix, which I don't think [the family had] known about previously. She [the sister] had sort of not wanted her family to be worried at that long distance so hadn't actually said too much about what was it about and then when she discovered what was happening here she told her sister. (09, gynaecological cancer, GP)

The following speaker talks of how his illness was communicated through the family. He explains that he had told one relative (a nephew) who went on to tell others about his diagnosis. This speaker was noted above to have been pleased that his cancer had drawn his family closer together. However, his daughter, living in America, is still not aware of his diagnosis or prognosis:

Oh I've got a big, family. [...] Do you want to know the truth? I don't want to inveigle my family. Right. [...] I mean to me the less people that know about it but they're, what do you want everybody to know what's wrong with you for? You most certainly don't. Because all they're doing is walking about with this 'oh I'm awful sorry to hear that. Ah no. Ah how do you feel?' [...] 'I would feel a lot effing better if you wouldn't keep coming over here and pitying me.' That's the one thing nobody wants. It doesn't matter what's wrong with you, nobody wants pity. [...] I wouldn't have told anybody, it was my nephew did that. He thought, 'aye'. But my daughter doesn't know, and I still haven't told her and I have no intentions of telling her, why should I? And the only reason, I'm just going to, I'll show you it. She sent me, I just got this [photograph], this morning. That's my grand-daughter and grandson right. (36, lung cancer, interview 1, patient only)

At the end of this extract he shows the interviewer a photograph of his daughter and grandchildren – citing them as a reason for not wanting to tell of his diagnosis, and the subsequent worry that would cause. In the second interview, this same speaker explains that he has still not told his daughter, but is now considering telling her next time she is in Scotland visiting, though he is unsure when this might take place:

Patient: Well, I don't know when, but hopefully it won't be in the immediate future, 'cause I don't want her coming here, its too recent and somebody would let the cat out the bag and I don't want that. I want to tell her myself on my own terms, I mean I had to put up with it because, ay, [nephew] had told my brother. But …

Interviewer: If it had of been up to you would have …

Patient: I would have said nothing. I would have just went on with it and left it as it, I only told three people. You know I told my best pal, I told [nephew] and I told his wife. [...] ignorance is bliss. But there's no way, I didn't bring her into the world to make her unhappy, so there is no way I am going to give her news. As I say.

Interviewer: So you are protecting her in a way?

Patient: I mean I've always done that anyway. <small>(36, lung cancer, interview 2, patient only)</small>

This participant was wary about how his daughter's visit might trigger someone disclosing the diagnosis with her. His role as a father appeared to weigh more heavily than his new identity as a patient, as he sought to protect her from learning of his illness. Other patients expressed wariness of how their illness might spark relatives to visit with a sense of urgency. The following speaker illustrates this and worries about upsetting her daughter and causing her to come back for what she perceives as a non-life-threatening illness:

Patient: [My son] has been quite concerned, been in contact by telephone. [My] daughter in Australia, em, a couple of years ago her father-in-law had a brain tumour, he lived in Elgin, and they came back for two years just to be nearby, to be supportive, eh, they were wonderful with him. He couldn't talk and he was in a very bad way. He died, em, and they went back to Australia. It was a real bonus for us to have them living nearby, she's on the phone or email almost every day but I do find that I can't tell her how much I'm missing her. [Both patient and partner crying].

Interviewer: I'm sorry, it's a difficult thing isn't it? That distance at any time really.

Patient: You know it's awful because I don't want to upset her. I don't, the last thing in the world I would want her to do is jump on a plane and come back here again and really the stage the children are at and everything she's just started working again and it just, anyway I don't think it's that important. It's not life threatening as far as I'm concerned at the moment. I'm going to get rid of this, em, you know deal with it and get back on with my life. <small>(53, breast cancer, interview 1, patient and partner)</small>

Summary

This chapter highlights the impact of cancer on relationships, partners and wider family networks. It also indicates the impact that relationships have on the experience of cancer. Within couples, and wider families, new ways of relating come about as a consequence of the illness; some of which lead to stronger, closer bonds, and others lead to troubled relationships and loss of intimacy. Life-cycle stages such as adolescence play a role in influencing the impact of cancer on family systems. In addition, geographical dispersion of the family mediate the experience of cancer, alongside strong positionings of 'parent' that effectively prevent people from disclosing their diagnosis to adult children, to protect them from worry. Indeed, patient and family relationships were often the vehicle for managing and understanding experiences of cancer. Overall this chapter has aimed to draw on the study's data to build a case for a need for systemic understanding of people affected by cancer, which must centralise the experiences of wider relationship networks in understanding the reach and impact of cancer.

Despite the clear message from these interviews that family members play a central role in the supportive care of people with cancer, policy directed at healthcare professionals to support and involve partners appears not to have always been translated into practice. This is discussed and debated in more detail in Chapter 10.

Chapter 4

Relating to professionals

Relationships between patients and healthcare professionals are important in the delivery of health care (Robb and Forbat, 2005). Indeed, in some fields such as psychotherapy, the relationship itself is considered the vehicle for recovery (Lambert and Barley, 2001). In recent times, relationships between patient and medical professionals have begun to change, with a shift in the power dynamic and expectations of knowledge, compliance and gratitude. Policy (Department of Health, 2001) has explicitly begun to position the patient as expert in their own experience, and subsequently as having a role in creating their own health and undertaking self-care (Lorig, 2002). Alongside this, family carers have become increasingly professionalised, which in turn alters their relationship with paid professionals (Forbat and Henderson, 2006).

This changing relational territory forms a backdrop to how people affected by cancer experience their interactions with healthcare professionals. Tracking such relationships is an important component of understanding the experience of cancer. Indeed, accounts of people affected by cancer underlined the importance of relationships with professionals as part of their experience of cancer and cancer care.

This chapter explores the accounts of how people affected by cancer relate to relevant healthcare professionals. This includes those working within primary care (such as GPs and community nurses), secondary and tertiary care (such as hospital-based doctors and clinical nurse specialists). Relationships with nurses and GPs are illustrated before describing the role of other professionals involved in the experience of cancer, with reference to follow-up care, the interpretation of communications and reflections on partnership working.

KEY ISSUES

- The overall experience of cancer care was dependent upon two features: the technical/medical care and the interpersonal interaction.
- The majority of people affected by cancer had very positive things to say about the nurses, doctors and other healthcare professionals they had contact with in their first year post-diagnosis. Professionals provided information and advice,

and held an important role of someone outside of the family connected with the experience of cancer.

- To most people affected by cancer, the idea of a healthcare professional being available, either in person or at the end of a phone, was very comforting. Trust was an important component of the relationship between patient and professional.
- General practitioners were described as being very busy, which was a feature often accompanied by an indication that they had not been in touch following a cancer diagnosis.
- Patients, at times, drew conclusions from how healthcare professionals interacted with them, for example being given time and attention was interpreted as a signifier of advanced disease and a poor prognosis.
- Patients felt that there was insufficient partnership working and care coordination between primary and tertiary care, meaning that there was a shortfall in providing an integrated systemic approach within and between NHS organisations.

Nurses

Clinical nurse specialists

Almost all the people in this study talked about the clinical nurse specialist (CNS) who was involved in their care. A couple of people acknowledged making very little use of their CNS, but in both cases, they had close relatives who were nurses, including one who was a Macmillan nurse. Family relationships and informal care thus sometimes took precedence over formal care.

People affected by cancer suggested that the role of CNSs was wide ranging. They were often present at the diagnosis, provided treatment information, helped with welfare benefit claims and often offered themselves as the preferred first point of contact when the person with cancer was in their own home. Several participants also spoke of how their CNS helped them organise funding for items that would help them take care of themselves at home, such as new showers. They also played a role in giving advice on making funeral arrangements. These functions were highly valued by participants.

Virtually all of the people who made any comment about their CNS did so positively using terms such as 'lovely', 'very helpful', 'brilliant', 'could not do enough', 'thoughtful', 'sensitive' and 'very approachable'. Approachability was highlighted by a daughter speaking of her mother's relationship with the CNS: 'And I think that says a lot for the type of person, or the role that she [CNS] plays, that you've told her [CNS] things that you haven't told your family as well, because she was so understanding' (52, lung cancer, interview 1, patient and daughter). Thus the CNS provided a critical role in enabling the patient to engage in conversations that she had chosen not to have with the family. The centrality of developing a trusting relationship seems clear in this speaker's account, referring to the 'type of person' but also the distinct 'role' of the CNS. As discussed in Chapter 3, people diagnosed with cancer relate to their families in particular ways when cancer enters their lives; at times patients draw relatives closer to them, and at other times patients wish to protect relatives from hearing the details of their illness. For the speaker above, it appears that the CNS fulfilled a particular role in enabling the patient to discuss the impact of cancer on her without troubling the family. The person with the diagnosis was thereby enabled to draw on the professional–patient relationship to help manage and maintain patient–family relationships.

Another participant indicated the importance of his relationship with the CNS, and how the care seemed dedicated and tailored to *his* needs. He was delighted that his CNS found time (and remembered) to telephone him with his latest test results before he went on holiday, enabling him to relax: 'Took my blood test one day, and she phoned me up the next morning to give me my results before I went on holiday just because the count came right down. She phoned me up just to let me know that before I went on holiday. And I thought that was a great touch, you know?' (04, prostate cancer, interview 3, patient and partner). Both he and his wife reported being very appreciative of the personal touch that this nurse had offered. This underscores how some professionals had shifted from treating just the disease, to treating the *person*, being mindful of how cancer fits in the broader context of their lives.

In the majority of cases, the CNS had provided their contact details and advised their patients that they were available at any time to answer questions or to assist with problems. This meant that care was provided round the clock and in a variety of locations. The following patient felt as though his worry was paramount to the CNS: 'Anything that I was ever worried about I phoned up [the CNS] and rather than wait for anything, she had me within a clinic within two or three days' (24, lung cancer, interview 3, patient and partner).

A CNS describes her role at the point of diagnosis as facilitating information exchange and subsequent diagnostic staging and testing, underlining how important the role is in facilitating relationships between professionals and patients:

> I went in with the consultant and he told her [the diagnosis]. I was just there, I sat through all that he told her and then he left the room and then I went on and spoke to [the patent]. I got details, I got all her personal details, her home phone number, and then I arranged for her to come back in to have some tests, to have the staging tests that they have done and I gave her my details, my contact details to phone me, and that was it. (12, breast cancer, clinical nurse specialist)

Further to this, another CNS described her role as reiterating elements of the diagnosis. This recognises an oft-named concern for patients that they forget what is said at the point of diagnosis.

Usually what happens is, we tend to sit in with them if we can, we try and sit in so that then we know exactly what's been said and basically reiterate it, if we haven't sat in, what we do is we see them after they've been seen by the oncologist and go over, say you know what they've said, we speak to the oncologist, you know, 'What's the plan?' and we go through it again and we go through the side-effects and things, we give them information, written information about the drugs, em, and we go away and, you know we say, you know, 'phone if you have any questions'. (39, colorectal cancer, clinical nurse specialist)

The role of the CNS was constructed by patients, partners and nurses alike as one where communication was fluid and the nurse was accessible and knowledgeable. Importantly, the CNS was seen to prioritise the person over the disease in their encounters, responding to them as more than just the site of a cancer. The following patient expresses this acutely in contrast to the doctor's approach to her: 'It was like she [the CNS] looked at the person with cancer, and he [the doctor] looked at the cancer within a person' (70, breast cancer, interview 1, patient only).

A couple of the people interviewed had never previously spent any time in hospital and the thought of doing so left them worried. The CNS facilitated a visit to the ward before her admission, which was well received, and was also ensured she was on the ward when the patient arrived for her treatment: 'I said "I've never been in hospital before," but really, they made it so simple, honestly. You wouldn't believe it, and then CNS came in and she was chatting to us and everybody was laughing and chatting' (61, breast cancer, interview 1, patient and partner). This patient's CNS offered her account of arranging the hospital visit:

The main worry for her was never having been in hospital before and being a bit worried about the hospital and all that kind of thing. So what I suggested was that she come up to see the ward and to see the hospital so that she could imagine where she was coming into and it wasn't going to be too dramatic, 'cause it's not, you know, it's quite a nice wee unit. (61, breast cancer, clinical nurse specialist)

Thus, the CNSs had a critical role in providing support to the patient and facilitating the fit between patient and hospital systems was as smooth as possible.

Ward nurses

Ward nurses provided a range of roles, including care during/after surgery and administering chemotherapy. Almost all people affected by cancer regarded ward nurses positively, using descriptions such as 'cheerful', 'exceptional' and 'lovely': The following patient carefully constructs the sensitivity required for changing wound dressings, including the time take by the nurse and need for delicacy: 'I'm impressed by the quality of nursing, it is very good … the care taken, you know doing things like changing dressings, which they can be quite brutal and it did involve time, but they were quite careful' (07, prostate cancer, interview 2, patient only). Other speakers also congratulated nurses on the care they delivered, even when people were feeling very unwell:

> They are really good, I couldn't fault them on anything at all, that time I really felt ill, I had to be at the doctor on Monday and by the Wednesday I was worse. So I phoned up [hospital ward], and it was one of the nurses who was there when I was there and she was really, really good, she told me exactly what to get. So when [my daughter] comes over she went to the doctor and got them, a few days and I was feeling much better. (52, lung cancer, interview 2, patient and partner)

> Again, I must congratulate the nurses. The nursing staff is top class, top class, they are really, and I've got nothing but the highest praise for these people. (46, lung cancer, interview 2, patient and partner)

Many people with cancer asked their nurses lots of questions about their cancer. One person who wished to have a 'wee chat' with a nurse had a conversation that lasted an hour. Giving of time was experienced as a very positive marker of care, as the following speakers indicate, explicitly referencing more junior NHS staff such as nursing auxiliaries:

> Once my wife and that went away I was really upset and an auxiliary nurse on the ward came in and spent half an hour with me, eh, and kind of calmed me down, really, really well, God, I mean, I can never thank that woman enough for, for coming in just having a chat. (28, colorectal cancer, interview 1, patient and partner)

> I got the chance in hospital, the second time I went back with the infection, of having a ward all to myself. There was nobody else in it for some reason, again probably understaffed and overworked. And that was the one time I managed to burst into tears and get it out of my system. Er, one little nurse passing, did notice I was balling my eyes out and kept chundering in to help. (40, gynaecological cancer, interview 1, patient and partner)

However, for some people affected by cancer the medical care itself was felt to be substandard, which was interpreted as an overall lack of culture of caring. Two people commented that their nurse did nothing when they said they were in pain. One woman with gynaecological cancer was in severe pain a week after surgery but felt that she was not believed by her nurse. A man with prostate cancer reported that he was told by a nurse that he had to be in 'real pain' before she would administer any analgesia. In both instances a doctor intervened and administered painkillers. This illustrates how powerful staff are in the provision or withholding of tailored medical care, and the subsequent impact this has on the person's overall experience of cancer.

Other negative comments concerned the variable ability of nurses giving injections:

> Some of the nurses know how to wield a needle and some of them definitely don't. I had one occasion where I, it was like I was being used like a pin-cushion, because they couldn't get the, they couldn't put it in right, you know, the nurse couldn't do it, I had it in there [indicates where the needle was put in], I had it in there, and eventually she went away and got another nurse who came in and pooof! Away in it went. (02, colorectal cancer, interview 2, patient only)

One woman with breast cancer found that she did not have anyone welcoming her when she arrived at the ward, and was given no dressings or painkillers after surgery. This woman had reacted badly to the surgery anaesthetic and had vomited causing her wound to re-open: 'They [the nurses] just didn't seem to react to that and get it fixed up for me you know, and I did get an infection in it' (53, breast cancer, interview 2, patient and partner). Poor relationships between professionals and patients, particularly when patient accounts of their experience were not believed, therefore led to unnecessary pain and distress.

Community nurses

Community nurses were seen by around a third of the people involved in this study. The most common reason for patients accessing community nurses was so they could assess and dress post-operative wounds or remove stitches. Other reasons included taking blood samples prior to chemotherapy, giving injections, enemas and general check-ups.

Most people affected by cancer were given contact details for their community nurse and advised to contact them as and when required. To many, the very act of the community nurse getting in touch with them, soon after their discharge from hospital, was very much appreciated, even if follow-up visits were not required. Health professionals recognised that people with cancer appreciated being contacted in the first instance. 'I think what happens with some GP practices is the district [community] nurse or the GP will phone just to say "Look, I'm here. You know this is my number. You know I'm not going to keep phoning you, but please phone me if you need me." And I think that's good practice' (05, breast cancer, clinical nurse specialist). People affected by cancer appreciated the flexibility and availability of community nurses:

> Even when I came home straight away I had the district nurse on to me, courtesy call, if I need anything she was quite willing to come out. (06, colorectal cancer, interview 1, patient only)

> I thought that was very good of the [community] nursing staff because there is a follow-up care there with this side of things. It wasn't just, 'Give us a ring'. (03, colorectal cancer, interview 3, patient only)

Some participants however had not been offered any support from community nurses. Slow healing wounds or ill-fitting catheters, for example, prompted these people to see their GP and it was only with this contact that community nurses became involved. One woman with a gynaecological cancer spoke of her attempts to not ask for help from community nurses, since she recognised this was a long drive from the GP practice to her home. However, though happy to change her own dressing, she had not been advised how to get more when she had used up the supply left by the community nurse and was shocked at the price of buying them herself. Her goodwill at saving nurses time seemed then to backfire with her feeling under-supported until she asserted herself:

> Nobody had told me that I could have phoned up the community nurses and got them on prescription, because they proved quite expensive. The next time they phoned I said I was not impressed at them having left me so few dressings. 'I'm trying to save you coming out here.' And ever since then they have been assiduously phoning me up to make sure I'm alright.
> (40, gynaecological cancer, interview 1, patient and partner)

A couple of people expressed surprise that they did not have any contact from a community nurse at any time after their discharge from hospital. People often expressed that even if they did not have urgent medical needs, the contact would have been welcomed as a general check-up. This contact would have been understood as a recognition that a diagnosis of cancer is a significant life event that requires support at different levels and different times. Thus, pure medical care in hospital was not sufficient on its own, and indicated a disjuncture between patient and family perceptions of the disease and professionals' views:

> I know they're very busy people, but I feel they could have taken five minutes just to pick a phone up, or, they're passing the door, you know, they could have just popped into see how I was, and, 'cause it was a big thing being told that you had cancer but, and then, as I say, they've never bothered since I've come home. (13, colorectal cancer, interview 2, patient only)

Thus, although there may be a precedent and belief that people are the experts in their own experience, this does not negate a need for practitioner-led interactions. People affected by cancer valued contact from nurses who could provide both medical and interpersonal support when experiencing cancer. This highlights an important element in working practices with CNSs and community nurses, regarding professionals' expectations about how forthright people affected by cancer would be in asking for services.

Doctors

Hospital doctors

Hospital doctors, including oncologists and surgeons, were typically discussed when describing the episode when the cancer diagnosis was given. Accounts of these doctors are peppered with emotionally charged descriptions of shock and devastation. Beyond those immediate responses, people spoke of a number of core attributes such as trust, accessibility and empathy, which were all highlighted as core competencies for hospital doctors. Each of these characteristics enabled people affected by cancer to forge a workable relationship, which would meet their needs.

Trust was important in two ways. First, trust acted to enable both patient and partner to take on board suggestions regarding treatment decision-making. People affected by cancer would often defer to medical expertise in following advice on which treatment programme to follow; having trust in their medical expertise was therefore critical. One patient said: 'You want to feel you trust the people that are specialists' (12, breast cancer, interview 1, patient only). Another remarked: 'I kind of trust what he, his judgment. I'm impressed with him' (07, prostate cancer, interview 2, patient only). Trust in hospital doctors was also expressed in messages to patients that any queries related to treatment should be directed to them, not GPs. Trust related to treatment decision-making is discussed in more detail in Chapter 9, in the context of confidence in the medical model.

The second component relating to the importance of trust in accounts was its interpersonal function in forming a positive ongoing medical relationship. Thus, as well as clinical effectiveness there was a strong desire for people affected by cancer to feel a sense of professionals' personal accountability. The following patient indicates how trust is a key component for her in being sure that she has been told the truth about her illness:

> There's a doctor always on duty and the nurse, they're always there. [But] you get different answers, em, and one, and this is part of the reason why I feel 'have I been told everything?' and it's very important to me, they should because of modern information eh, you can get so much information now, [I] can't cope; if I think you're hiding something from me, it breaks my trust. (31, gynaecological cancer, interview 2, patient and partner)

For other patients, their relationship with hospital professionals was built on previous negative experiences, which framed and informed their current experience. One woman plainly explains this, having been given false hope for her mother's illness:

> [The doctor] gave me hope a week or two before my mum died, which was false hope, she would have been better just not saying nothing at all. Do you know what I mean, but no, I'm working, she's working with me but I know I can look at my files at any time so, I'm trying to build my trust up ... that's why I don't like going to the doctors. (26, gynaecological, interview 1, patient only)

Trust was also, at times, built upon professionals' reputation: 'I do trust them, I trust her [the consultant] because I know from years ago from friends who've had her before, that's she good' (34, prostate cancer, interview 2, patient only). Trust was considered to be related to doctors' specialist knowledge; thus they had an important role in instilling hope for people:

> *Partner:* Right from the start [surgeon] said, there was an 80% chance that [Patient 01] could get better, em, I think that made us both feel very positive about it, and from then on we just always tried to look on the positive side and [consultant] did say to you about your positive attitude.
>
> *Patient:* Aye, that's right, so she did. (01, colorectal cancer, interview 2, patient and partner)

Accessibility was an important element to feeling in touch with professionals in the hospital. Patients expressed pleasure and surprise as consultants at times gave them mobile phone numbers with which to contact them. Empathy was a further core component to how people affected by cancer related to hospital doctors. Although many positive examples were cited, some speakers constructed notions of physicians who struggled to develop an empathic relationship:

> Well, I think that there is … I don't think the consultants really have been in a charm school enough, when you're …. erm, when you're suffering, when you get the news of cancer from the …. from the consultant, and then within a week or so, you're then transported up to the [hospital] and you're still reeling from this and it's a surreal situation and it so … I would feel that when you go in, I don't think the way … the consultant spends enough time just with you, just quietly talking through it and sometimes give the impression of being a little bit off-hand as well, and just eh … You know just doing a bit more in the way of … of … of that side of things that I think … Terribly matter of fact. (03, colorectal cancer, interview 2, patient and partner)

Participants expressed their understanding that doctors were busy, but neverthe-less liked it when there was a personal, not purely clinical, element to their relation-ship. Some patients took responsibility themselves for transcending the ascribed positions of patient and doctor:

> It's nice to not be so impersonal as well, and I mean I know she's a very busy lady but, and she was always very sort of business like and I thought, I knew she'd gone on holiday, so I just said as we were leaving one day, 'did she enjoy it', and she said about her girls. So, but it was nice, because you cant always just be too business-like, em, I think you need a wee bit of a personal touch …. [I can understand why they] don't become personally involved, because you could, you've got to cut yourself off from your patients, I can

understand that, but at the same time, I think she appreciated the fact that [the patient] recognised her as not just a doctor, but as a person with a life outwith the hospital. (01, colorectal cancer, interview 2, patient and partner)

Relationships with hospital doctors were strained when it became clear to patients that they had not prepared for the appointment by familiarising themselves with the treatment and tests that had gone before, which led to frustration and disappointment: 'She obviously hadn't read the notes, just as much as she maybe should have, you know' (01, colorectal cancer, interview 2, patient and partner).

Other hospital staff

Aside from oncologists and surgeons, a range of other hospital professionals were involved in people's staging, treatment and follow-up appointments. There was a great deal of praise for the range of NHS staff within hospitals, and many patients mentioned junior and non-medical members of staff who had played a role in making the experience more tolerable: 'Every person in the [hospital], even to the wee lassie, God bless her, that gave me a cup of tea in the morning, everybody was brilliant. Unfortunately, the hospital itself, needs a lot of work done to it. But that's totally irrelevant' (01, colorectal cancer, interview 1, patient and partner).

Negative comments were also made about care received from non-nursing and non-medical hospital staff. One radiographer was described as 'a bit nippy', and many other patients felt that the communication they received was lacking. One breast cancer patient was distressed at the poor way in which clinicians related to her. At one point she invokes her professional self (as a former nurse) and questions the evidence base of their practice:

At one point they all went, they all went away in to the room and I just suddenly thought, 'God it's gone awful quiet', and I was just lying there exposed on a, a thing and I, and I moved my head and they all come running back in. 'We told you not to move, we told you not to move!' ... and I was like, 'But yous all went away and left me,' and she says, 'Well, we found that if we tell people that, that we're going, then they're more likely to move,' and I was just like, so I wish I said to her, 'And can you give me a reference for that please? Because I've never heard it.' Everything that I mean, we do communication skills all the time through nursing ... explain what you're doing. (70, breast cancer, interview 2, patient only)

For this speaker, the personal experience of cancer was in the context of her identity as a (former) nurse which enabled her to re-examine her own understanding of healthcare practice.

For many of the above participants, even when medical care itself was clinically accurate, the interpersonal element was lacking, which meant that the overall experience was not positive.

General practitioners

General practitioners were identified as exemplifying both the best and worst aspects of care that people received. Many described their GPs as 'very supportive' and 'excellent'. Some people kept in touch with their GP by phone, and had regular appointments with them throughout their cancer treatment. Keeping in touch was a hallmark of how people affected by cancer viewed a positive relationship with primary care. There was a clear view that GPs were very busy and this got in the way of forging the kind of relationship that people affected by cancer desired. Several people with cancer appeared reluctant to express dissatisfaction with their GP, and it was often their relatives or friends that described what was felt to be lacking.

When contacting a GP about cancer or treatment-related symptoms, many people affected by cancer reported that GPs were unable to provide answers to their questions. People were therefore often redirected to hospital staff who had specialist knowledge: '[GP] admitted that, you know, "This is not my area of expertise, you really need to go back and see, you know, the surgeon and discuss at the hospital"' (05, breast cancer patient, interview 2, patient only). The partner of one person diagnosed with lung cancer also reflected on levels of expertise in primary care: 'He's a bit inexperienced with oncology, with the drugs and things, because when you go for a prescription when you had your infection, he doesn't know and he was scared just with the contrary medications and mixing them … but he quite admitted that' (52, lung cancer, interview 2, patient and partner).

Keeping in touch

General practitioners that initiated and maintained contact following a cancer diagnosis were praised for their support, however, this was variable between GPs. One woman with breast cancer described the role of her GP as superb: 'So again, he said "If there's anything else," come back to see him as soon as … every time go round and see him, he always says that to me, he asks me how I am and everything, oh yeah, he really has been superb' (09, breast cancer patient, interview 2, patient only). Most people with cancer received a phone call from their GP, or in some cases, the community nurse, soon after their cancer was diagnosed or after surgery. This was always appreciated and expressed recognition of caring for them as an individual as well as the disease:

> And [GP] said 'I've just had a fax about you from [hospital]', and I went, 'oh, gosh,' and she said 'I just wanted to phone you up to say I'm here if ever you want to come in and talk to me' and she said also, 'The other doctors, we'll all know about you' … I thought it was extremely nice of her to phone up, it really was, to pick up the phone at half past six at night. (10, breast cancer, interview 2, patient only)

Often the initial phone call included the promise of regular contact, which sometimes did not occur, which lead to disappointment:

He did say to me right from the outset, 'We'll keep in touch, you can come and see me, and then we'll have a telephone call in between,' [...] but he's never got in touch or anything, and when I did actually make an appointment he decided to phone [...] and I got the impression he was in a terrible rush, I told him what I wanted and he said he'd get that ready for me, but he didn't ask how I was, not once, just a quick rush, 'That's fine, I'll get that for you', bang down the phone went. I thought well, that's contrary to what he was saying earlier on. (19, prostate cancer, interview 3, patient and partner)

This feeling of the GP being terribly busy was articulated by a large number of people: 'And the GPs, they're so busy that I'm just a name. As a matter of fact, I think I've never had the doctor I signed on with, when I first moved into this area here, I've never had her since! And that was fourteen years ago. I've always had different doctors' (46, lung cancer, interview 3, patient only). Another person felt neglected on not receiving a further follow-up phone call from their GP: 'obviously you're just a reference number' (29, colorectal cancer, interview 2, patient and partner).

After treatment finished, the hospital-based healthcare team ceased contact with the patient and their partner. This was often experienced as a difficult time for people with cancer, leaving them feeling that they had lost a significant form of professional support and the potential for a reassuring relationship. Often there was an expectation that primary care physicians would fill this role. When GPs did not meet this expectation, people reported feelings of isolation and 'being in limbo'. There were expectations that GPs might be in touch via the telephone, as the following partner expresses: 'There was support there when she went in but as to, kind of like, them ringing her or anything like that, I know it might be a bit intrusive for them to keep in touch with people, but there wasn't really a great deal going on like check-ups or anything ...' (05, breast cancer, interview 3, patient and partner). The following partner expresses a similar sentiment, expressing a feeling of disconnect from services. 'But I mean, the aftercare ... the authorities could have helped out more, I feel, but it's like who do you speak to when you get like an automated system or an answering machine? It's like there's no real people out there any more to speak to' (06, colorectal cancer, interview 3, patient and partner).

One person described a lack of awareness at her local surgery and the subsequent difficulty experienced attending to have stitches removed. Asked if she had had contact with her GP, she replied:

No, it's never mentioned ... I mean, they do the repeat prescriptions for tamoxifen, so they presumably have a vague idea what it's for ... I went to have the stitches out ... the practice nurse had no idea what it was for ... I suppose it's quite interesting because to start with she was being quite 'right and you've got stitches to come out have you?' And she said 'Where are they?' So I told her. She said 'Oh' ... the attitude changed radically in a very short space of time ... they must know, because I mean, letters seem to zoom back and forth and everything ... (27, breast cancer, interview 3, patient and partner)

As with speakers who had expected follow-up contact with community nurses, there was a feeling that a lack of contact from the GP practice was indicative of an overall lack of care and a sense of an inadequate professional relationship.

Perceptions of priorities and GP busyness

General practitioners were widely viewed as extremely busy professionals. Many participants recognised GPs could be quick and effective and that this wasn't necessarily at a cost to the patient, but became an organising principle in how people prepared themselves for appointments. One couple joked about the hectic pace of their GP: 'His ten-minute consultations are ten minutes and he moves through the Health Centre complex ... he should really be on a skateboard. It would save his legs [laughs]. He goes like mad' (40, gynaecological cancer, interview 1, patient and partner). One couple described their GP's approach as well paced and unrushed: 'Never, never rush you [...] he goes over anything, he checks up on his screen what's been happening and checks what ... and again, he asks us if there's anything you want to ask about' (18, prostate cancer, interview 1, patient and partner). Being given time was therefore constructed as a signifier of good care for this couple. In contrast, other people expressed their reservations about how long they felt they could speak with their GP. Despite having many questions remaining about their prognosis and likelihood of disease recurrence they felt rushed in their appointments:

> *Patient:* The disease itself reacts differently in different people I believe so, eh, but I would like to hear it from a health professional what are the chances of this recurring you know, em, if it is going to spread will it spread to the breast, will it spread to the liver, just will it spread? You know.
>
> *Partner:* We hear it wasn't in, I can never get the names of these things, lymph ...
>
> *Patient:* Lymph nodes, they apparently are clear. So that seems to be a good sign.
>
> *Partner:* Seems to be a good thing.
>
> *Patient:* I'd like to be able to balance it up a bit more in my own mind.
>
> *Interviewer:* More information. Do you ask your GP questions about ...?
>
> *Patient:* He's, I think this is the problem with the whole medical profession at the moment everybody is pushed to the limits. Eh, I don't know how long a GP is supposed to give you, I think it's a minimum of ten minutes. I felt three to four.

Partner: Three to four minutes, I've watched it on the clock. (40, gynaecological
cancer, interview 2, patient and partner)

There was also a fear of not wanting to become 'a nuisance' to GPs thereby putting
in jeopardy the relationship people affected by cancer already had with them. One
individual accepted his GP's idea of keeping in touch via the telephone as opposed
to face-to-face consultations to cut down on consultation times, clearly positioning
this as related to the GP's important and busy role beyond the primary care clinic:
'He teaches at the medical school and he's the local medical officer of health as well.
So he's quite tied up. But he said he would look at arranging … you know, meetings
and then alternate meetings on the phone' (19, prostate cancer, interview 1, patient only).

Participants had sometimes felt that their needs had been taken seriously as GPs
occasionally had suggested that people with cancer inform the receptionist they
'were one of her cancer patients' to allow prioritisation. The experience of cancer
was thereby constructed as significant for GP, patient and receptionist. This led one
patient to reflect on the need for such catastrophic news to feel like a priority: 'He's
been really nice, it's terrible that you have to had cancer before they seem to have any
time for you, but he really is nice' (52, lung cancer, interview 2, patient and partner). Thus, in the
context of GPs being viewed as very busy, important work was being done by both
people affected by cancer and professionals in negotiating the changed relationship
with primary care. GPs were viewed as occupying a central position in providing
supportive care for many people with cancer.

Interpreting communications and behaviours of health professionals

Interpreting the communication of healthcare professionals, regardless of whether
they were nurses, doctors or other practitioners, was critical in how some patients
related to staff. Patients and partners would attribute meaning to interactions that
were unintended by the healthcare professional. One CNS summarised one of her
experiences, and this perhaps sheds light on why official job titles were not always
used by staff and were often poorly understood by people affected by cancer:

> My post was initially funded by Macmillan and one of the doctors, I always
> remember, at clinic had said, 'I'll get the Macmillan nurse to come and see
> you.' And the woman just point blank refused. But I did catch up with her
> a few months down the line and she always remembered that day. And she
> said to me, 'You know, it wasn't that I didn't want to see you,' she says, 'It
> was because he said Macmillan.' She says, 'That freaked me out.' She says,
> 'I couldn't handle that.' … Now they just introduce me as 'the lung sister'.
> (63, lung cancer, clinical nurse specialist)

In the same vein, two men with lung cancer did not welcome a referral to the community nurses. One of these men was concerned that having a specialist cancer nurse come to the house would imply that he was not coping, and he did not wish to give this impression to those around him. Thus, even contact with health professionals was deemed a communication too far for some patients.

Although the attentiveness of nurses was generally regarded very highly, a couple of people found such attention to be suspicious. One patient in particular, reflected on the close attention he was getting, and made him wonder if he had 'got to that stage yet' of not being capable of looking after himself. Other people shared similar worries that staff interest in them signified bad news regarding their diagnosis or prognosis: 'There was quite a few nurses around and they were all exceptionally nice, which in a way, you think, oh my goodness, what's going to happen, because they are actually, you know, falling over their feet to be nice to you, so you know that something's, somebody's going to tell you something you don't want to hear' (27, breast cancer, interview 1, patient and partner). Likewise, facial expressions (however inadvertent) were interpreted as a non-verbal communications of bad news: 'I knew fine when I, when I saw, it was the nurse who was just attending to me immediately after, I knew fine by the look on her face, I just knew there was something wrong' (38, colorectal cancer, interview 2, patient and partner).

The above quotations highlight the importance of the ability of health professionals to communicate with patients and partners in realms and arenas of life that are sensitive and require compassion. An obvious issue requiring good communication skills is talking about death. Some patients for instance, had discussed with health professional their wishes around end of life care. The following extract illustrates how people affected by cancer interpreted specialist professionals' relative ease at talking about such issues, with reference to resuscitation:

> *Partner:* The staff are just, they're just so tuned in and they're just so sympathetic and empathetic and you know, you just have this feeling that they're completely genuine, there's a transparency there which you just don't get … in a, in a gen med ward
>
> *Patient:* And also, they're more comfortable speaking about, it sounds awful, cancer and death
>
> *Partner:* Yeah uh huh, yeah, yeah.
>
> *Patient:* And, and one of the things that came up em, was the 'Do Not Resuscitate' form that exists. And they brought that up in the Marie Curie em, where that would never have been discussed I'm sure in a general ward. But it was one of the doctors we had been dealing with, who very em, diplomatically em, you know spoke about lung cancer patients. (69, lung cancer, interview 3, patient and partner)

For this couple, the medical context of palliative care compared to general medical wards opened up valuable opportunities for discussing death. The diplomacy of the specialist doctor enabled a useful conversation to occur, focused on end of life care for people affected by the same tumour.

Inter-organisational whole systems working

Patients and partners reflected on their views of the interactions between components of the healthcare system and its impact on them as 'service users'. The multiple job titles and role that nurses occupied contributed to confusion for patients and made it hard for them to know how to relate to professionals.

Many people affected by cancer referred to the CNS as a Macmillan nurse, whereas others had done the reverse. In some instances, it was not entirely clear from the interviews conducted for this study which one is being referred to. As noted above, often professionals made a conscious decision to not label themselves in order to manage how they were perceived, and were consequently related to, by patients.

A CNS described the role of different nurses, and offers her explanation in relational terms, suggesting that certain nurses take a backseat, to enable the relationship between patient and chemotherapy nurses flourish:

> When patients go and have their chemotherapy, we kind of take a step back because the chemotherapy nurses take over because they see them more regularly, so we tend not to hear from patients and then it all sort of starts up again after that, we tend to sort of see them again … they build up a relationship with those nurses for that period of time we kind of take a step, because you know having too many people gets, you know, is just a bit intense so we sort of, I'll probably take a bit of a step back. I mean, obviously, if he phones and he's got queries, then we'll deal with it, but I would imagine what'll probably happen is that they have numbers for the chemotherapy units and they'll phone there. (39, colorectal cancer, clinical nurse specialist)

Although this change in which healthcare professional takes the backseat may be clear and intuitive to the nurses involved, reports from people affected by cancer revealed that it was not effectively communicated to them. This lack of clarity created problems for some people affected by cancer, leading them to feel uncertain who to approach with queries or problems. The description above frames the withdrawal of CNSs to be an informal arrangement, so confusion is not an unexpected side-effect for patients.

One patient reported confusion over who to contact and under what circumstances. As with contacting GPs the idea of avoiding being seen as 'a nuisance' was important:

I was under the impression was I could only phone her if I was ill … You know, if I, if I saw any of the symptoms of the chemo, I mean, like, er, then I would phone her. I didn't know that she was a support nurse … plus the chemo nurses up there are really busy. You know, there's no way that you want to bother them [laughs]. (42, gynaecological cancer, interview 3, patient only)

A similar view was expressed by another individual: 'You don't quite know who's in charge, is it the GP or is it the consultant?' (32, colorectal cancer, interview 2, patient and partner). Various people expressed views of poor organisational issues across services. The following speaker, for example, refers to both primary care and specialist nurses as lacking the requisite skills: 'If there was something going wrong I don't feel my GP and my breast care nurse will pick it up. You know, because I don't have confidence in them to be proactive enough to sort something out' (12, breast cancer, interview 3, patient only).

Mixed messages regarding who patients should contact resulted in confusion and irritation for some people affected by cancer. A call to one professional would at times lead to a string of recommendations of other, more appropriate, people to call. One man contacted the hospital regarding a chest pain and was 'a wee bit surprised because they told me to phone my own doctor' (46, lung cancer, interview 2, patient only). He then described being referred to the hospital following side-effects from the medication prescribed by a locum GP and said his consultant, 'was not amused that the hospital had told me to phone my own doctor', but he added 'that's between them and her.' Thus, it was not uncommon that people affected by cancer felt as though they were holding the information and services in their heads and negotiating services' views of other parts of the system. Taking ownership of information and continuity often fell into the hands of patient and partners. This was evident throughout diagnosis and treatment, and was noteworthy for many participants in this study for alerting the GP to their health status: '[The GP] phoned me and says "can you tell me why you was discharged from the hospital? What were you in for?" And I said "Heavens above, I've been in since the end of January with cancer"' (20, gynaecological cancer, interview 2, patient only). Examples of such missing communications were all too common, leaving the patient responsible for passing messages from hospitals to primary care. People expressed disappointment at having to provide this link role:

It's this joined-up thinking, whenever I've had to contact him, I've been the one who's had to fill him in with where I'm at, you know, how I am and everything, and I think that's disappointing. (14, breast cancer, interview 2, patient only)

There is always a lack of communication between hospital and the GP, because when I saw [consultant] he said 'You've started on the tamoxifen', and I said, 'No,' I hadn't and he said 'Oh, you should have started it by now, you should have started it by now'. So I got on the [GP] surgery and they get all huffy because they haven't been told […] it's awkward because you are stuck in the middle and if communication were better it would be a lot easier. (27, breast cancer, interview 2, patient only)

For people who had a change of CNS or GP during treatment, there was a clear feeling of lack of continuity and a loss of a potentially valued lengthy relationship. 'The only thing that would make a great difference to you, if you could just get to see one doctor rather than seeing a whole load of doctors' (06, colorectal cancer, interview 3, patient and daughter). For some people the lack of communication was considered to have serious medical consequences. For one individual a serious infection resulted from a communication failure, which the patient was shunted into taking responsibility for:

> When the notes came through there was no mention of this infection in them. The GP who saw me at the time tried phoning [consultant] to find out more about it but couldn't get hold of him or his secretary. And said to me, 'Oh [Patient 40], why don't you just phone him from home?' and I thought about it and I thought maybe I imagined it, so I didn't follow it up 'cause I know health professionals are at the end of their tether, they're at the end of their ropes with the NHS. (40, gynaecological cancer, interview 1, patient and partner)

Healthcare professionals also identified with these accounts of un-integrated care systems. One CNS identifies a lack of computerised notes as the reason for not always being up-to-date with patients' treatments. The emphasis on pushing communication is placed at the feet of GPs: 'We are not in the loop to see what, you know, there's no computer link between community and ourselves to see what's happening out in the community, but I'm sure if the GP had been running into problems then he would have referred [Patient 20] back to the ward' (20, gynaecological cancer, clinical nurse specialist). A GP offered a different account, reflecting more closely, like the people affected by cancer had reported, that the patient often held the information: 'The problems we often have is the delay in communication between hospitals and us sometimes, but that's not a disastrous thing and it's better at some clinics. It's always difficult when the patients come to you and say "this, that and the other thing has happened"' (54, breast cancer, GP).

The lack of joined-up working between NHS silos was evident in some people's ???? accounts and illustrates the clear shortfall in the ability of the health service to work in a way that was respectful to the person's individual needs: 'I just think it was more, it was a kind of process and you were kind of part of a process. I got a feeling it was a kind of sausage factory … you know … I should be feeling elated that it's all over, but you kind of feel as if, almost like I'm having my worries now' (12, breast cancer, interview 3, patient and partner). This quotation appears to indicate that the process of treatment ('a kind of sausage factory') was suboptimal. Although the outcome in terms of clinical disease seems to have been successful, her exclamation that she 'should be feeling elated' is telling of the shortfall between physical treatment and the overall patient experience.

Summary

Overall, healthcare professionals were seen to be providing a good level of care, with nurses contributing to a solid culture of caring, and ensuring that core physical, emotional and informational needs were met. Despite this, criticisms did arise. Notably, GPs were identified as having a lack of specialist knowledge, which is problematic for people affected by cancer who expect them to provide support around diagnosis, prescribing medication, symptom management and providing aftercare and follow-up. The relationship between people affected by cancer and healthcare professionals played a role in mediating the overall experience of cancer. The development of a positive relationship between professionals and people affected by cancer weaves its way through people's accounts of their experiences. Without a positive alliance, care was felt to be impoverished and fall short of meeting the needs of people affected by cancer.

This chapter exposes opportunities for refinement in the provision of care between tertiary and primary care, suggesting that partnership and joint working is not yet meeting basic expectations, such as coordinated information sharing between services. Aiming towards a greater level of systemic working and provision of outpatient treatment will necessitate a shift in how GPs support people affected by cancer. Thus, policy directives will have implications for community health practitioners to provide more support to both the patient and their partner or those acting as informal carers.

Chapter 5

Relationships with others who have experience of cancer

Someone is diagnosed with cancer in the UK every two minutes, and over the lifetime one in three people will develop cancer (Cancer Research UK (CRUK), 2009). It is therefore, not surprising that most people who are diagnosed with cancer know someone else who has a direct and personal history of cancer. This may be a friend, neighbour or colleague who is a current or previous patient, or a family member of someone diagnosed with cancer. In this chapter we describe the role that these people play for those who are diagnosed and living with cancer in the first year following their diagnosis. We also describe the ways in which other patients who are also recently diagnosed and being treated for cancer relate to one another and interact. In doing so, we develop our understanding of cancer within the context of relationships wider than the family and professional networks.

Interactions between people with a history of cancer and those who are newly diagnosed are often informal, and instigated by people affected by cancer as opposed to being nurtured and encouraged by health and social care professionals. The informal characteristic of these relationships and interactions can be contrasted to support/ self-help groups run by voluntary organisations. These groups may have informal beginnings, but once established become routinised and sometimes subsumed into formal organisations. Their purpose is largely to provide support for and by people affected by cancer; the common feature of these groups' members is their direct and personal experiential knowledge of cancer.

This chapter illustrates how important such experiential knowledge is for people who are personally affected by cancer. Such knowledge is awarded a different and higher status than understanding gained through professional clinical trainings.

KEY ISSUES

- People with cancer have been through similar experiences and therefore belong to the same 'club'. Being a member of this club means being able to support others with cancer based on direct and personal experience of the disease, which is based on experiential knowledge.

- Patients are providers of information to other patients about diagnosis, treatments and symptoms.
- Listening to another patient's experience of cancer can be a strategy for coping. It can make a patient put their own problems into perspective because they learn that others are worse off. Talking with other patients can make people realise that how they feel is not unusual or abnormal.
- People recently diagnosed with cancer seek out, or are offered, information from their friends and neighbours who act as an important source of advice as a consequence of their experiential knowledge.
- Friends and neighbours may put a positive spin on having a cancer diagnosis and stress success stories of people surviving cancer. Some people with cancer however do not necessarily wish to hear about these 'survivors'.
- Friends and neighbours provide practical assistance as well as information. This is because some people who have had direct and personal experience of cancer wish to help others who are also affected by cancer.
- For people with cancer who are in paid employment, colleagues can also influence the ways in which they relate to their experience of cancer. Knowledge of symptoms and treatments from work colleagues is another information source.

Relationships in context: belonging to the same club

People who are ill and use health and social care services possess a specific kind of knowledge that is derived from direct and personal experience, which we refer to in this chapter as experiential knowledge. The term can be traced to the concept of experiential learning that was developed in the late 1950s. John Dewey (1963) who influenced the development of a model of experiential learning (Kolb, 1984) and reflective practice (Schon, 1983) developed a philosophy of experience. His thesis is that knowledge and learning comes from direct participation and is achieved through reflection upon everyday experience. We use the concept of experiential knowledge in this chapter to suggest that people affected by cancer are active knowledge creators who construct meaning *in situ*, and in doing so have something unique to offer other people, including other patients. Although the concept has been used as an analytical device to understand the nature of self-help/support groups (Borkman, 1976), we use it as a framework for understanding informal relationships between people affected by cancer.

Our study suggests that people who have been through a similar experience (that is, a diagnosis of cancer) develop relationships with each other that are different to those with people who have no direct personal experience. As one of the people with cancer in our study put it, people who have been through a similar experience belong to the same club: 'I had some fascinating conversations with people about that, all different ages, all different cancers, and you have, you're in a club if you like, you know you have a common denominator ...' (69, lung cancer, interview 2, patient and partner). In this chapter we interrogate the significance of this club and inferred membership criterion. People who have been through a similar experience know how it feels. We suggest that having a very similar experience enables individuals to speak, listen and relate to one another in ways that others are not in a position to do. It illustrates how cancer can affect relationships (by opening up new relational opportunities) and how new relationships can affect perceptions and experiences of cancer. As the following quotation shows, talking to others with cancer can be important:

> *Interviewer:* Is it easier talking to somebody who's already had cancer than somebody that's not?
>
> *Patient:* Well I, I found, and this, I mean I was at a function ... and one of these guys who's a friend of my wife's father had come across ... and he speaking to my wife's dad and he's oh you, you know, 'I wasn't well last year, I, well I had cancer' ... so I perked up ... and I spoke to this guy and I, I felt so much better after talking to this guy ... I got such a lift just from speaking to this guy and his attitude again and it was, so I've, you can share things with people, that have had it, 'cause you can say, 'oh did you get this and did you get that,' whereas I can say to my wife, 'I got this and I got that,' and she, obviously she knows I've, I've had it but she doesn't really, she doesn't know, I don't think that anybody that hasn't done chemotherapy can imagine ... so I, you'd end up, I'd end up falling out with my wife, saying 'you don't realise how I'm feeling' ... and she's saying 'but I do realise how you're feeling 'cause I'm affected by this as much as you are.' (28, colorectal cancer, interview 2, patient and partner)

The quotation illustrates that family members, including wives, husbands and partners, may not always appreciate and recognise the value and significance of experiential knowledge that comes from direct and personal experience of cancer diagnosis. Although family members are in many respects sharing the experience of cancer with the patient (as described in Chapter 3), this is not the same as having a similar experience of being diagnosed with cancer.

Often, others who have had a personal and direct history of cancer are the first to openly discuss cancer with a recently diagnosed person. This can be perceived as genuinely helpful to those who have recently had similar treatment:

> *Patient:* One girl in particular just in the village and she had, had problems with her bowels she hadn't had a malignancy but, in other words, she'd been for the same sort of ...

Partner: Surgery

Patient: Surgery, and she volunteered information, she was the first to say 'look, honestly you couldn't be in better hands' and she was very, very positive, then there was people that we'd met on holiday … my wife came back off the phone … you know practically singing because this lady had said, 'look my partner has had the very, very same experience, and he was very positive about it, again the same people he was concerned with and he's come through, so you tell your husband that, not to worry, be positive in your thinking'. So I've had a lot of that thing from friends, from good friends, but not just airy fairy, speaking in generalities, people who have actually experienced what we're going through just now and that was a big help. (38, colorectal cancer, interview 1, patient and partner)

Having experience of being diagnosed with cancer uniquely positions that person so that they have the knowledge to support others in a similar position. Having had cancer, there is a belief among participants that this can give the person strength that enables them to provide support which otherwise might have proved too emotionally demanding. One woman who had recently been diagnosed with cancer explained why she thought that people who had been through a similar experience were able to provide support to others:

Interviewer: And is there something special or different about somebody that's gone through it? In terms of support, or other than a health professional or something?

Patient: Oh I think so, you are a much stronger person if you've gone through something, aren't you? Than someone that hasn't. I mean you take bereavement, if somebody has been through bereavement they can comfort a person that's just facing bereavement for the first time. They can tell them how to cope with it, can't they.

Interviewer: Is that something you would be interested to hear, how other people had coped?

Patient: Well if they said 'well this helped me or that helped me', Yes, I think so. (10, breast cancer, interview 1, patient only)

Another participant who was interviewed just after receiving his diagnosis said that he would have welcomed the opportunity to talk to someone who had been through the same experience. He said that people with cancer may be more willing to ask another person with cancer questions that they do not feel able to ask healthcare professionals. In this way, lay relationships are privileged over more tricky relationships with healthcare staff. He also implies that it may inspire hope because it shows that people survive cancer. He appreciated that it was not possible to speak to someone prior to surgery because he was treated as an emergency and had surgery within twenty-four hours of admission:

I think I would like to see ... people would go in who suffered from it themselves and would have a chat ... And yes I think, if it were possible, I think you know, your healthcare people do a good job, your surgeon does a good job, but somebody just coming in and saying 'hello, I have been here, I have got cancer, I've em' ... somebody to come and say 'look at me I'm still breathing. Have you got any questions? How are you feeling?' that sort of thing. Questions that you might not ask your consultant ... yup, from that point of view, somebody could come in who was not a health professional. (03, colorectal cancer, interview 1, patient and partner)

Below, are more examples of the relationships that people with cancer within the first year following diagnosis forge with others who share a similar experience. We first focus on their relationships with other patients and then go on to describe their relationships with friends, neighbours and work colleagues who also influence their experience of cancer. We highlight how cancer is experienced within relationships between those with experiential knowledge derived from direct experience of being diagnosed with cancer.

Relating to other patients

A significant source of information for people within their first year following diagnosis is other patients who are undergoing similar treatment. Clinics and wards are places where people with cancer meet and communicate with one another and are the locations where relationships between patients are forged. Patients tap into each other's experiential knowledge in these settings. One of the advantages of these settings is that there are a range of people at different stages in the care pathway; some are still undergoing investigations whereas others are undergoing treatment.

The people with cancer who we interviewed not only told us that they obtained information from other patients but some of them also recounted how they had acted as a source of information for other patients. For example, one man with prostate cancer who was undergoing treatment explained that he was able to describe what happened to him to two other men who were having investigations prior to treatment:

I met quite a few. There were people came in for the same problem. And they were going through the assessment when I was going, this was on the Monday I went for my operation. I had the other two gentlemen who were on the ward with me who were up for assessment, which I had had three weeks previously. So I could tell them what I went through, you know. So they had to come back in for the treatment. So we all had a talk about it and the various problems they had and we were all similar, you just know all similar. (04, prostate cancer, interview 2, patient and partner)

Not every patient, however, wishes to learn about the experience of others or to interact with other patients. One woman, for instance, did not want to know about the plight of others because it detracted from being able to cope with her own problems:

> They were all very nice and we all took our sweets and 'would you like a sweet?' and they are all very chatty but there was just this one person in particular. Em, I just thought: I wish she would just be quiet. But fortunately that was her last treatment so she was lucky. A terrible thing to say, but I really don't want to know anybody else's business. I've got enough to cope with. (25, gynaecological cancer, interview 1, patient only)

And another individual stated a preference for not conversing with others while in hospital awaiting treatment because hearing about other patient's problems rocked his confidence:

> I was sitting in the day room and there's a telly and again I was playing the game and there's a guy getting chemotherapy, and again I'm, I'm not one oh these guys that likes to share my problems with everybody, so another guy comes in and he sits down, 'are you in for chemotherapy?', 'aye', 'first time?', 'aye', 'oh, it's a lot oh shite, I've been ill, and I've had this and I've had that'. Go away, you know what I mean? Sorry, but I ignored the guy and then he slammed the wall, 'do this and then crap, can't sleep at night, ah murder, crap.' [...] it wasn't doing any, my confidence any good. (28; colorectal cancer, interview 1, patient and partner)

Our study suggests that men and women may use experiential knowledge as a strategy for supporting each other differently. Relationships for male and female patients are perceived as different, and interviewees presented this gendered division as an unproblematic assumption. One man who was diagnosed with colorectal cancer reported a perception that men may mention to each other that they have been diagnosed and treated for cancer whereas women discuss their experience in more depth. The following extract constructs this as a joint understanding of the role of gender between the male patient and his female partner:

> *Partner:* Maybe breast cancer, women within, will all talk about it.
> *Patient:* Not men.
> *Partner:* Men, no. I think women are more open about different operations that they get done to themselves, you know, or what their spouse has done, I suppose it's like prostate cancer and things like that you know em, there's not a lot of men talk about that either and I don't think even when you talk amongst themselves particularly
> *Patient:* No really, you know, maybe mention it, but I mean, it's not talked about or discussed about.

Partner: Uh huh, whereas a woman, as you know, will go in to all the details.

Patient: Whereas men will sit with a few boys and having a drink and just discussing different things, things come up when you're talking, you know. (39, colorectal cancer, interview 1, patient and partner)

A gender dimension to interactions and conversations between people with cancer may also be evident on hospital wards. One woman who was diagnosed with cancer perceived that women with cancer discussed their treatment and how they felt whereas she did not believe that men did the same:

> Yes, I know she was so scared when she came in so it was a couple of us in that ward tended to cuddle her up. Tell her you know, 'Come on we're all scared this is horrible, its not nice what's happening to any of us but we're all here for each other' and we were. It's amazing thing. And I've heard people say that in the men's ward, the men don't talk about it, they don't discuss their treatments they don't discuss how they feel. The women discuss how they feel, which I think is a great thing. (40, gynaecological cancer, interview 1, patient and partner)

Although we would not want to convey an essentialised understanding of gender, the participants in this study did construct an idea that gender did have relevance in mediating people's experiences and relationships with others.

Conveying information about diagnosis, treatments and symptoms as described above are not the only motivators for interacting with other people with cancer. Listening to another patient's experience of cancer can be used as a strategy for coping with a life threatening condition. This seems to be particularly the case if the other person's experience is worse than their own. One woman said that it made her feel better when listening to other patients because it made her realise that others were in a worse position than her. She describes conversations (conflabs) with others that she was reassured by:

> Oh yeah. From the staff as well as the patients as well. We all have a conflab or patients have the conflabs and it really brightens you up when you come in here and you speak to some of the other women. I think I am badly off and then I speak to some of them and I think 'my God, how dare I feel like this?' in many cases. Some of the women what they've gone through and are going through. (09, gynaecological cancer, interview 1, patient only)

Listening to another patient talking about a similar experience of cancer can act as reassurance because it notifies them that their experience is not uncommon. One patient said that she did not feel so stupid feeling scared and crying after she had heard that other women receiving chemotherapy were also emotional:

Patient: There was one night I was lying in my bed and I just … yeah I did have a good sob to myself. There was one of the patients in there the first night I came in, she said she did that one night herself. She said 'yes', she said 'I just bottled it up. Well not bottled it up' she said 'I came through here and just lay in my bed and sobbed and sobbed'. She said 'it's just a part and parcel'. They all, the patients say the same thing.

Interviewer: So that's a good camaraderie, a good support?

Patient: Oh yeah I mean the first morning I went through for my chemo-therapy I was quite emotional, but I think as well, because it's the first time there was a fear of the unknown, being emotional and my God what am I going to go through. Scared of what I was going to go through and everything. So I remember saying to the clinical nurse specialist 'I feel so stupid', cos she came through for me and she took me through to the chemotherapy room and she said 'don't be silly, it's ok.' And then after the first chemotherapy and my radiotherapy that day I came back through here and the nurse talking to a couple of girls who were in for different reasons altogether and I told them about being emotional and they says 'we would have been in the same way,' probably been crying their eyes out and then I didn't feel so stupid. But I know it's not … to feel stupid … it's just the emotions going through us. (09, gynaecological cancer, interview 1, patient only)

Patients awaiting surgery on a hospital ward can also ease the anxiety of others by creating a relaxed atmosphere through chatting with one another about other issues besides cancer and laughing. One woman spoke warmly about her time on the ward:

Patient: I can't believe how wonderful it was … this woman said 'oh I've baked some banana bread' you wouldn't believe this. So she brings out her banana bread and she says 'oh I've got some biscuits oh would you like digestives or tea, oh I'll have some of those, oh I've got this, I've got this.' So we're all sitting there, like [laughs] what was …

Partner: [laughing] It was surreal

Patient: You know everybody just chatting, nobody's talking about cancer or anything. We're just, and all introduced ourselves and I'm so and so and so and so. (61, breast cancer, interview 1, patient and partner)

Relating to friends and neighbours

People with cancer who participated in this study drew on the previous experience of friends and acquaintances who also had a direct and personal history of cancer. People recently diagnosed with cancer seek out, or are offered information from, their friends and neighbours who act as an important source of advice as a consequence of their experiential knowledge. Within the first year following diagnosis the information that people with cancer in our study wanted from their friends and neighbours related to details of diagnostic investigations, treatments and symptoms/side-effects.

The information could be gleaned without the friend actually realising that the person quizzing them was in the process of, or had recently been diagnosed with cancer, but this was unusual. One man, for instance, said that he questioned a couple of his friends at the bowling club who had been diagnosed with the same type of cancer in the past before letting on that he had also been diagnosed with prostate cancer:

> *Interviewer:* Ok. Tell me about … you've obviously talked to some people that you know at the bowling club. How did you broach that?
>
> *Patient:* They weren't turning up for games, some of them, they weren't turning up to play their games and they were asked what was wrong? And they started to tell us, you know. There are two or three. In fact one was so fed up with the treatment that he was getting that he is away back to Italy to see a specialist in Italy.
>
> *Interviewer:* So they've had prostate cancer before you got your diagnosis?
>
> *Patient:* Yeah.
>
> *Interviewer:* So you were aware of them? So, you've told them that you've got …
>
> *Patient:* No, I haven't told them.
>
> *Partner:* No, you haven't said anything to anybody else.
>
> *Interviewer:* They don't know you've got it yet?
>
> *Patient:* No, no. But I was quizzing them about their treatment [laughter].
>
> *Partner:* Just to get an idea.
>
> *Patient:* What to expect you know [still laughing!].
>
> *Interviewer:* And has that been helpful?
>
> *Patient:* I think so, I think so. (04; prostate cancer, interview 1, patient and partner)

Friends and neighbours, when providing information, are usually aware that the individual they are talking to has recently been diagnosed with cancer. They often provide this information because it has been requested by the individual with cancer. The information that is given by a friend or neighbour before the individual undergoes an investigation or treatment can run counter to the actual experience. This may be due to the friend or neighbour deliberately underplaying the pain or other symptoms that may have to be endured because they do not wish to frighten the individual. One woman who was due to have a mammogram, for instance, was led to believe that it would be relatively painless because a friend had informed her that she would be fine, but found this not to be the case: 'I had been told by a friend that I'd be fine, because I had plenty of breast tissue, it doesn't work that way, I think some people, it's, it's not fine for anybody' (21, breast cancer, interview 1, patient only). It is, however, understandable that friends and neighbours wish to put a positive spin on having a cancer diagnosis and stress success stories of people surviving cancer. Some people with cancer appear to welcome positive examples because they find it reassuring and it is what they wish to hear. People with cancer may not deny that others die from cancer, but they do not necessarily wish to hear about them:

> *Interviewer:* How have you found talking to other people about their experiences? You said you know some people …
>
> *Patient:* Yes, … first woman I mentioned it to, em, I had to say I was going to be late because I was going to a hospital appointment and it all came up that I was going to get this breast lump looked at and then she, you know, I said 'I'm sure it's benign. Oh well, I hope you get on okay because I had the, you know I had a breast lump and this was about twenty years ago' and there she is large as life. So that was very reassuring and the other person I spoke to she had gone through it all about two years ago and I, you know, she was fine. So the positive ones are always good to hear and then I know of odd cases and you see there's, I think I've heard of people at work who've been diagnosed with breast cancer and in my mind I've just written them off thinking 'Oh well, we won't see her again' sort of thing you know? And I'm thinking people will be saying that 'Oh God, [participant's name] she's got breast cancer, well that's her' sort of thing. You know. And I know there are tragedies and I know people who have died from breast cancer or are dying, em, but that's been with metastases and all the rest of it and I just think well I'm lucky it was small and it was contained and blah, blah, blah. […] you only want to hear the good stories and not the bad and most of the people I know have only been telling me the good stories thankfully. (55, breast cancer, interview 1, patient and partner)

Friends and neighbours who have undergone a similar experience may help to put the impact of a cancer diagnosis and treatment-related symptoms into perspective for the individual with cancer. One woman who was coming to terms with losing her hair as a consequence of chemotherapy was able to reframe the impact of hair loss after being visited by a friend who had undergone similar treatment in the past. It led the woman to conclude that hair loss was a small price to pay for being alive:

> Well sometimes, I know I'm alright just now but I know that maybe after my next chemo or my chemo after is when my hair starts falling out. This is when I know I'm going to be down. Because I've always tried to kind of

look half decent and put make-up on and, but, em, I know this is going to be awful. But I have a friend who went through exactly the same this time last year, but she had breast cancer, so she went through chemo, so she's been over and spoken to me and she said it's not really that bad, your hair grows back and it's a small price to pay for your life isn't it? (25, gynaecological cancer, interview 1, patient only)

This example shows how relationships with other people who have a similar experience can help patients to contemplate the meaning and impact of treatment and weigh-up whether treatment-related side-effects are worth the price of staying alive.

People affected by cancer who have recently been diagnosed often have internalised ideas of cancer and its treatment from accounts they have heard long before their own diagnosis. In this context, the information about investigations and treatments may not have been deliberately downplayed or given in such as way as to alleviate others' fears. For example, one woman recalled what she had been told by a neighbour who worked in a radiography clinic thirty years ago about radiotherapy. This recollection frightened her to such an extent that she decided to find out more about radiotherapy from the internet:

> *Interviewer:* It sounds like you've been doing a bit of information seeking yourself if you've been going on the web and looking at things.
> *Patient:* Yeah, well I had to because like I told you, when he said radiotherapy em, I had a neighbour thirty years ago who at one point had the job of putting the pessaries inside women who had cancer of the uterus and she got the job because she was sterilised and her family was complete … and she used to tell us about the horror stories about people's insides being burnt 'cause it was a radioactive cobalt piece of metal used to fire inside these poor ladies and it burnt their bladders and their bowels and their intestines and it you know did horrible damage to their immune systems and when it comes to their breast tissue they put little pellets in the breast … and people were badly scarred and burnt … plus the fact you don't want to go through the rest of your life suffering, you know, horrendous pain and, I mean I wasn't going to have bladder or bowel problems, but there's other ones, so em, the clinical nurse specialist had like said, that wasn't so, so I decided to go on the net and find out. (21, breast cancer, interview 1, patient only)

This quotation highlights how previous relationships and experience of cancer shape how people newly affected by cancer relate to, and construct meanings about, their own recent diagnosis.

As well as being the recipient of information and support from friends and neighbours, an individual with cancer in turn acts as a provider of information about investigations and treatments because they now have direct and personal experience that may be of use to others. One individual in our study informed another person living in the same village as him about how radiotherapy has impacted on the tumour:

> I've got a friends who's, she lives in the village and she's got cancer of the oesophagus, and she's just gone in for radiotherapy and she didn't know that the tumour would carry on reducing … em, I was given that information, but she's, apparently not been given that information and eh, when I told her about that, she says, 'oh, I never knew that, no' … but she was quite pleased to know that because I had, could pass on the information.
> (02, colorectal cancer, interview 2, patient only)

Friends and neighbours can also provide practical assistance as well as information, driven by a desire to help others who are also affected by cancer. One of the ways in which they can do this is to drive others to hospital for treatment, which runs in parallel to formal hospital transport services. Although some patients may use these formal hospital transport services, others rely on informal support from friends and family to get them to and from appointments. One woman in this study had to remain in hospital during treatment and required a lift home each weekend. Friends and acquaintances who had been affected by cancer themselves rallied round. One of her sister's friends offered to pick her up from hospital; the patient perceived that one of the main reasons that he offered this help was because the volunteer had a personal experience of cancer:

> I get a female family friend, takes me on Monday and a male, well he was actually, my younger sister was at college and he got friendly with her through there but his wife has had I think I'm not sure if it's a double but she's had a mastectomy for breast cancer. She's been there herself so he again, they can totally understand what's going on and that and he's coming in. He'll take me home on Friday's, so it's, as I say we've had offers left, right and centre from people offering 'just pick up the phone and let us know and we'll soon come in for you, no problem.' (09, gynaecological cancer, interview 1, patient only)

A further way in which friends are invoked in accounts of cancer is associated with the notion that one discovers which relatives and friends can, and cannot, be depended upon. The following quotation draws from this idea and offers a cautionary tale:

> An old lady that I knew … well I know … well I see her today for the first time since I've had my chemo, when I told here I was gonna have to have this operation and that. 'Well' she says 'I'll warn you now' she says 'I've had breast cancer' she says 'I had radium treatment after it' and she says 'don't

rely on your friends' I says 'what do you mean?' she says 'all my so-called friends, as soon as I took ill; they desert you, they won't come near you or nothing' she says 'I used to have to come from my radium treatment and get in my car to go and do my shopping 'cause I had no family.' And she was right!! (06, colorectal cancer, second interview, patient only)

Thus, although friends were routinely identified as helpful and supportive, drawing often on their own experiential knowledge of cancer, this was not always the case. As the last speaker identifies, with no family to provide support, friends may provide some other avenue of hope. The rationale for friends being unavailable and 'deserting' people newly diagnosed is not explicitly articulated, but may be explained with reference to the wider socio-cultural space in which cancer is experienced, which is discussed in Chapter 9.

Role of others: work colleagues

Circles of friends and neighbours are not the only people who can provide information and support to people with cancer. For people who are in paid employment, work colleagues can also influence the ways in which people relate to their experience of cancer (this is the focus of Chapter 6). Work colleagues, like friends, can act as examples of surviving or dying from cancer or they can be the bearer of information because they possess experiential knowledge as a consequence of their direct and personal history of cancer. One man explained how the death of two colleagues, who had been diagnosed with cancer, spurred him to visit his GP to investigate his own symptoms. The deaths of people in his work context made him aware of the importance of receiving an early diagnosis before evidence of metastatic disease. When he first noticed symptoms, he went straight to his GP:

Yeah, eh, I mean I suppose I don't go to the doctor very often so I was quite happy getting these tests, I mean biopsies weren't the most pleasant of things, em, but there's actually two colleagues who worked in the school here in the physics department who both died of prostate cancer ... So I was quite aware if it wasn't caught early what the implications could be so I was quite happy to get things checked out. (07, prostate cancer, interview 1, patient only)

Thus colleagues (alongside family members, as described in Chapter 3) play a critical role in the timely diagnosis of cancer, acting as informal spurs to get symptoms formally investigated.

Treatment is an important topic of conversation between work colleagues who have been diagnosed with cancer, particularly in discussing how to manage treatment-related symptoms. This information is highly welcomed and valued prior to commencing treatment. One individual had spoken to a colleague who had been diagnosed with another type of cancer and found it invaluable. The information that he was given by the other person was practical and focused on how he would feel after chemotherapy and how he should manage his pain:

> He was chatting things about it. He had said to me that it is not, you feel some days that you feel you are a little bit better, but it's the next day, you are better than I was yesterday and you do, you can feel yourself eventually getting better. And he had said to me 'anything they give you, take, because even although you might not feel in pain, if you don't take it, a few hours later it wears off what the previous stuff you gave, and you start to feel the pain, so just keep on taking it. If you don't put it in your mouth just put it at the side so you can take it when you do feel it.' It was very good to actually talk to him about it, somebody that had gone through the same, something, maybe not the same but something similar. (02, colorectal cancer, interview 1, patient and partner)

Colleagues can be a welcome source of information if they are able to share good news such as offering examples of people surviving cancer: 'One of the girls in the work, her father he had bowel cancer twenty-four years ago and he's eighty-four now … so, I mean, you ken what I mean that's a good, that's a good illustration for me, I, I'd focus on that rather than reading, oh there's a guy died of bowel cancer' (28; colorectal cancer, interview 2, patient and partner). The same individual, however, was also aware through his workplace of others who had died in hospital, which made him fearful:

> I had, had a situation one of the girls at my work eh, this year, who'd went in for a minor operation into hospital eh, and they had cocked it up, she was supposed to be in and out in a day, cocked it up and eh, she was in the hospital in intensive care for three months and died, so instantly I'm thinking, anything to do with major surgery's going, I'm, I'm a goner basically. (28, colorectal cancer, interview 1, patient and partner)

Examples of deaths from cancer in the workplace created atmospheres of worry, and contextualised people's own relationship with the disease.

Summary

The focus on the role of non-familial relationships offers a dimension for understanding how the disease is experienced within relationships which are often overlooked.

People with cancer relate to each other in ways that are unique because of their experience of being diagnosed with cancer. In the words of one participant, they belong to the same club. Experience is thus a key context, and influences how people with cancer relate to others and the role that others can play. Through this experiential knowledge they are able to offer information to others about how diagnosis and treatment actually feels. This information is valued by people recently diagnosed with cancer. They are in a position to reassure and help others cope with their diagnosis and treatment. Alongside providing information and advice, people affected by cancer often provide practical assistance. Their own personal experience is an impetus to supporting others in a similar position. Their very presence can act as an example to others and can be a beacon of hope. However, as other chapters in this book have demonstrated, other people who do not have direct and personal experience of a cancer diagnosis play an extremely important role in supporting the individual with cancer. Family members, in particular, share the experience of cancer.

Chapter 6

Work and employment

Given improvements in cancer survival (Verdecchia *et al.*, 2007) the number of people of working age living with cancer in Europe is likely to increase. In the UK, approximately 500,000 people under the age of sixty-five have been diagnosed with cancer at some point in their working lives (Cancer Backup *et al.*, 2006). A systemic approach to understanding the experience of cancer should take cognisance of relationships with others within contexts deemed significant by the individual with cancer. One such context is the workplace.

Examining employment through a relational lens, which focuses on interactions between people with cancer and other people, is uncommon. The traditional focus of employment research is measuring the amount of time that people with cancer are absent from paid work and identifying factors that predict absenteeism. Research carried out predominantly in the United States indicates that most people with cancer remain in, or return to paid work upon completion of treatment (Spelten *et al.*, 2002; Steiner *et al.*, 2007).

Recent research has examined reasons why people with cancer return to work, as well as barriers to, and facilitators for, their return. These descriptive studies show that people return to work for a range of reasons including financial (Kennedy *et al.*, 2007; Main *et al.*, 2005), because it provides them with a sense of self-worth (Main *et al.*, 2005), and because they have a desire to return to a sense of normality (Kennedy *et al.*, 2007; Main *et al.*, 2005). Research highlights some of difficulties encountered at work due to physical and cognitive impairment (Main *et al.*, 2005; Maunsell *et al.*, 2004) and suggests that employers and colleagues can facilitate continuation or return to work by supporting a decrease in hours or changes in their work responsibilities and schedules (Main et al., 2005). Finally, research suggests practitioners do not provide sufficient information or support about employment-related issues (Kennedy *et al.*, 2007; Main *et al.*, 2005; Maunsell *et al.*, 2004).

In this chapter, we argue that a systemic approach is an important contribution to the practice, by highlighting the significance that others can play in supporting people with cancer in the workplace.

KEY ISSUES

- The impact of stopping work during the onset of a life-threatening illness such as cancer can come as a shock to people who have always been in paid employment.

- Healthcare professionals can encourage people with cancer to realise that they may be able to continue in paid employment despite the illness. They can play a role in allaying the 'guilt' that some people with cancer experience when taking sick leave.

- Alongside physical reasons for not being at work, for example being in pain, people also require time to recuperate and adjust to the impact of cancer. Cancer is more than a disease entity; it is life changing.

- Some people with cancer imagined how colleagues would relate to them in their current physical state, and cited this as a reason for not wishing to be at work.

- Senior managers and human resources influence people's experience of cancer in and out of the workplace. They can facilitate people's access to sick pay through clear communication, signal that the priority is the patient's health and well-being, and ease a successful return to work. Our study highlights examples of helpful and unhelpful communication and process.

- Work colleagues can relate to people with cancer in a positive manner by explicitly showing that they care about the patient's health and well-being and by helping them to manage the impact of cancer on their ability to do the job.

- Not all people with cancer return to work following a cancer diagnosis. Two main reasons for not returning are that the person is too ill or the person is nearing the age of retirement. Irrespective of the reason, the transition out of work leads individuals to re-negotiate their relationship to paid employment.

- Policy (as described in the introductory chapter) acknowledges the role that partners play in a patient's care. However, this can be restricted unless the partner's employer facilitates this caring role by enabling them to have time away from work. Permitting absence from work to care varies from workplace to workplace and is an area of negotiation because policy and procedures are not always in place or clearly understood.

Relationships in the context of employment

A systemic approach, which situates people's experiences with cancer beyond the clinical setting, aptly draws attention to the relationship between an individual and paid employment. Occupation is a principal means through which many people develop and express their identity (described in more detail in Chapter 7), providing a sense of purpose and structure in day-to-day lives. Occupations are 'More than movements strung together, more than simply doing something. They are opportunities to express the self, to create an identity' (Christiansen, 1999: 552). The impact of stopping work during the onset of a life-threatening illness such as cancer can, therefore, come as a shock. One woman with cancer said it was difficult stopping work because 'I'm not used to it, I mean I've always worked, I've always been out working, if I'm not working I'm always doing something in the house or out the house' (08, breast cancer, interview 1, patient only). Another woman with breast cancer said that stopping work 'Was quite a shock, really, when you've not had any blips for thirty years. Psychologically it's a very odd feeling to not be at work' (14, breast cancer, interview 1, patient only). Health and social care professionals have a role to play in supporting people as they temporarily or permanently exit paid employment. They can encourage people to realise that they may be able to continue in paid employment despite the illness. They can allay the 'guilt' that some people feel about being on sick pay:

> They did say in the hospital, 'Please don't go giving up your job.' I think it was the clinical nurse specialist that said that, 'Please don't go handing your notice, or such like,' she says. You know, which people can do because they just, you know, don't know what's going to happen. She says, 'Just see what happens', you know, 'It's ok to be on a doctor's sick line', 'cause I've never had a doctors sick line in my life until last time, the other day there, the other week there, em, so I felt better when they said its ok, 'cause for someone that's never normally off work, so you feel quite guilty. (69, lung cancer, interview 1, patient and partner)

One of the reasons that some people with cancer give for not being at work is because they did not feel capable of doing the job. That is, they give a functional reason. One patient said 'It would be a bit of a waste of time going back to work today and then maybe a couple of days time, saying, "Oh my God, I cannot do this because I'm sore"' (08, breast cancer, interview 2, patient only). Another woman with breast cancer, whose work was physically demanding, returned to work once she was strong enough and the pain had gone. Initially when she went back to work she did not carry out certain tasks, reporting that she experienced a slight weakness in her chest. She said 'I've always stated quite clearly that I'm not coming back until I'm able. I'm not going back when I know I cannot do my job' (05, breast cancer, interview 2, patient only).

Alongside physical reasons for not being at work, for example, being in pain, people also require time to recuperate and adjust to the life-changing impact of cancer. A clinical nurse specialist expressed this clearly when she said that people with cancer may 'technically' be able to go back to work but they need time to deal with the impact of cancer as a 'life-changing event':

> One of the things I really do believe could be better is, instead of taking the patients, we ... give patients lots of support at the point of diagnosis,

through their treatment and then off they go, which is fine, you know … instead of just discharging them after their treatment would be to have some kind of formal teaching or group sessions whereby they could actually learn about what's happened to them and get some advice about how to readjust their lives for the future, because having a diagnosis of cancer is actually a life-changing event. And you, whilst you're thinking about surgery and chemotherapy, you're not usually dealing with those other issues, which is how you're going to live after it … Because you know, technically, they could go back to work, then, the treatment's finished, but that's often when they stop and take stock and think, 'Goodness, what's happened to me in the last few months, the last year.' (21, breast cancer, clinical nurse specialist)

This clinical nurse specialist locates the impact of cancer in relation to a person's whole life, therefore perceiving cancer as more than a disease entity; it is life changing. The following quotation (a patient of the previous speaker), draws our attention to the wider impact of cancer on life:

Well, I, I'm hoping that when I go back to the doctor on Thursday that she will let me stay off sick a little while longer, I feel I need some recovery time, some time off work that isn't for going for treatments if you know what I mean. That's all I seem to have done … endlessly, is up and down to hospitals and people sticking needles in me or doing things to me, and I'd like just a wee while to recover, to find my feet, get a bit more hair… I want this time off just to recuperate, like I said, the time off, when I'm not looking to go up for treatment, you know, that I can just get myself together, gather my strength up and then go back and think, 'that's it I'm back to work, I'm healthy, life's normal, you know, that's it done and dusted.' (21, breast cancer, interview 3, patient only)

Some people with cancer imagined how others in the workplace would relate to them in their current physical state and gave this as a reason for not wishing to be at work. They expressed concerns about their physical appearance and the impact of this on others. The following two examples draw our attention to relationships within the work context, and the role that cancer plays in shaping identities. A man with colorectal cancer had stopped working since his treatment because he had a colostomy bag. His job involved visiting people in their own homes and he did not think it appropriate to do this while he needed a colostomy bag. He said: 'Well you couldn't really go to somebody's house with a bag of rubbish hanging off your side' (01, colorectal cancer, interview 2, patient and partner). One woman did not like the way that she looked and therefore stayed off work: 'It was just such a shock. I don't think I could have … And I didn't look right at all, I looked awful. Well, down here I thought I looked awful, em, but they've [employers] been excellent, they've been really, really good … I don't know when I'll go back to work' (25, gynaecological cancer, interview 1, patient only). These two speakers may have been physically capable of functioning at work, however, they did not wish to return because they were concerned about the impact of their altered appearance on other people. This relational component was also significant in how people perceived their working lives with senior managers in the first year following diagnosis.

The role of others: senior managers and human resources

Senior managers and human resources (HR) influence people's experience of cancer in and out of the workplace. Indeed, employers have a legal obligation to support people with cancer to return to work. They can facilitate people's access to sick pay through clear communication and ease a successful return to work. Some people with cancer in our study recounted how they had contacted HR to find out about their entitlement to sick pay:

> They can't just say, 'Oh well, you've got cancer we can't take you back,' you know they've got to find a way and they're very good but I don't know how that, what role that would be. But I said to you [name of partner] yesterday, today 'I'll have to try and not worry about that 'cause that's not my problem, that's, the you know, the organisation to find that one out.' (69, lung cancer, interview 1, patient and partner)

Further, this patient highlights that HR may have to discuss with them the subject of death in service:

> I went into HR last week and asked them, for the first six months you get full pay, em, and then after that it goes like half pay if you like it goes down to 'cause SSP [statutory sick pay] kicks in more than your, your employer and then after a year there isn't pay, you just go on to sort of whatever allowances that your local authority government give you, yeah, so I enquired about that, I also enquired about my pension because there is a lump sum, for you know death in, in service. (69, lung cancer, interview 1, patient and partner)

However, many people with cancer in our study were not totally clear about their entitlement to sick pay, their rights or welfare benefit entitlement. One woman with cancer for example, was not sure about her entitlements because she had never had a sick line before. A man with cancer was also vague about his sick pay entitlement because when he contacted personnel they were unclear. Several people with cancer had negative experiences with their employers when organising sick leave and their return to work. One woman with cancer was advised by her doctor to plan a phased return to work rather than immediately going back full time, however, she ran into difficulties trying to organise this with her employer. She reported feeling bullied into returning to work:

> I had a phone call on Thursday morning, my new manager ... and she wanted to know where I am in this illness and when I'm planning to come back, and I have to have an official meeting to discuss all this, and the only good thing about it is I went screaming to the Union because she's supposed to do a letter first but she said 'No', and I told her I couldn't really afford to come through to Perth and it wasn't, you know, and you know, it's a bit hard to say, 'Yes, I will be well enough to meet you on the twenty-first or the twenty-third,' or whatever day she picks, because I don't know, so what I've got now is her, I'm waiting for the letter to say that she's coming here, let her use her petrol up. And she's bringing human resources, but I did kind of feel that I'm getting bullied to get back to work, I've had six months off, you know, I've had, this is me, you, 'You have had twenty-six weeks absence this year now', and that's counting my hospital appointments as well, it's not all been, you know, some of them are just the odd day for hospital, so that's me, 'Twenty-six weeks, get back to work, girl.' (21, breast cancer, interview 3, patient only)

The reference to this speaker's manager as being 'new' may be of significance here, as it signals perhaps an idea that they have no former relationship from which they are operating. For people with lengthier relationships with employers, the situation had been different. Some participants in this study had only praise for their employers. A man with cancer suggested that he take his annual leave entitlement to attend hospital for appointments, but his boss said that he should just take time off. He calculated that he had had around six weeks off in total including two weeks while an inpatient and four weeks while he received radiotherapy as an outpatient. Another man with cancer said that the directors of the company that he worked for offered to pay for a private room while he was in hospital so that he did not have to have a bed on a ward. The directors of the company also contacted his wife to see if she needed support of any kind. A woman with cancer described her employer's response to her situation as 'very good'. She worked for a large public sector organisation that transferred her onto 'special' leave as opposed to sick leave, which meant that she would still need sick notes, but would not lose her pay. She described her workplace as like one 'big family', clearly invoking the importance of interpersonal relationships in workplace experiences of cancer. Her boss, whom she had known for years, visited her at home after her diagnosis to see how she was. She also kept in touch with colleagues and met some of them for lunch because she missed the office banter. One woman with cancer found her boss's response to being told that she would be having six weeks off work very reassuring. Her boss said: 'I don't care, as long as you're better at the end of it' (08, breast cancer, interview 1, patient only). This employer clearly indicated that the main priority was the patient's health and well-being.

The role of others: work colleagues

Work colleagues can relate to people with cancer in a positive manner by explicitly showing that they care about the patient's health and well-being and by helping them to manage the impact of cancer on their ability to do their job. Several people with cancer praised the response of colleagues who showed that they were thinking of them and cared. A man with cancer received various gifts during his absence from work including a basket of fruit, and a bottle of champagne when his results showed that he was 'all clear.' He also received plenty of text messages, cards and phone calls. This type of support, alongside the support from family and friends, helped him to get through something that he said he would never like to go through again.

> The support of colleagues is also important when the individual with cancer returns to work. This is because they can support them by helping them to manage the impact of cancer on their ability to fulfil their role. People with cancer may welcome the opportunity to be able to phase their return to work by slowly increasing their hours and they also appreciate changing the way in which they worked, for example, not lifting heavy items or working less hard. They needed the support of their colleagues to be able to make these adjustments. A woman with gynaecological cancer explained how she had the support of her colleagues: 'So I think the only way to build it up is, if I, I've got a great office, so I just need to say "I'm tired" and, and I won't need to worry' (42, gynaecological cancer, interview 3, patient only).

Colleagues acted as a source of support if they had experience of cancer themselves. We discuss the role of others who have direct and personal experience of cancer in more detail in Chapter 5. Here, we provide a couple of examples of the role of work colleagues. Familiarity with cancer among colleagues was felt to be a huge support. A man with cancer said that three other people in his office also had cancer, which meant that they were able to empathise and understand what he was going through. One of his boss's relatives also had colorectal cancer and so understood why he was not able to work. A man with prostate cancer said that his boss 'understood' because he had also had prostate cancer: 'He's familiar with it all. He's been through it' (04, prostate cancer, interview 1, patient and partner). One woman with cancer compared notes with a colleague about their experiences of cancer, which, according to this woman's relative, gave her an 'enormous boost' (09, gynaecological cancer, interview 3, partner only). However, talking with others about cancer could also be stressful. This woman found talking to a colleague stressful because it was near to her first anniversary of being diagnosed, a time point which she felt was a significant but stressful milestone:

Last night I was a wee bit tearful at work, because talking to one of the girls, that was her sister that's been through the skin cancer, it'll soon be a year and I think that's what's coming up as well, it'll soon be a year and I think that's telling on me, I think, I got scared when ... I don't know why, I just started getting jittery and scared and I thought 'look, stop it, you'll be ok.' I just want to get the year past with and I think its building up to that and I know a lot of it is psychological as well. (09, gynaecological cancer, interview 3, patient only)

Re-negotiating the relationship with paid employment

In this study some people remained in work following their diagnosis, and throughout treatment. These individuals did not have to contemplate returning to work or reflect on the ways in which their social and economic status could be put in jeopardy as a consequence of cancer. A man who was diagnosed with prostate cancer, for instance, only took time off work to attend appointments for scans. He did not have any adverse symptoms that would warrant time off, although many of his colleagues were amazed that he had not been off work because they all assumed that he would feel ill. One woman with breast cancer only had a week off, which was during surgery, but then returned to work while she was receiving radiotherapy. For these individuals there was minimal need to renegotiate contractually with work.

Some people however, having taken time off work for treatment did not ever return to their job. Two main reasons for not returning were ongoing symptoms/side-effects, or the proximity to an expected age of retirement. Irrespective of the reason, the transition out of work leads individuals to renegotiate their relationship to paid employment. This transition is a process and leads individuals to reassess their position and identity as someone in or out of paid employment.

Some people with cancer in our study who were near their age of retirement decided to retire early following the diagnosis. These people, therefore, not only had to contend with a diagnosis of cancer but also with retirement, which was often a major life-changing event in itself and signals entry into a new and significant life-cycle stage of older age. A man with cancer whose job involved public speaking, presenting to audiences and supporting people on a one-to-one basis, decided to retire early because he had lost confidence. He reported that he could not concentrate and found his type of work too emotional. His doctor was concerned that he was retiring early because the doctor perceived that he was 'giving up the ghost'; the GP encouraged him to consider staying at work for another few months given that he reported feeling physically well. He, on the other hand, wanted to prepare for retirement as soon as possible: 'I think I would rather say now, "That's us, that's the end of our chapter." I'm not going back' (03, colorectal cancer, interview 2, patient and partner). Yet, the decision to retire early was not made immediately, but took time. The reason for this decision was because retirement for him was 'life shattering.' He, therefore, not only had to manage a diagnosis of cancer, but also giving up a job he had previously enjoyed.

People who are or become too ill within the first year following diagnosis also renegotiate their employment situation. Pain, shock, sickness, tiredness and loss of strength, confidence and ability to concentrate were some of the overriding reasons why other respondents also did not work during treatment. During chemotherapy a woman with lung cancer had given up any expectation of returning to work because she was very ill. Her consultant, however, suggested that she could go back at some point because she was responding well to treatment. In the context of several hospital admissions, blood transfusions and debilitating symptoms such as a high temperature, sweats, pain, low energy, vomiting, diarrhoea, and rashes, this suggestion inspired her to start to plan her return to work. For example, she discussed with practitioners about reducing pain relief medication that made her drowsy and was contemplating a phased return, part-time hours and a different role at work. Despite this, she was redefining her place in the social world by submitting to the inevitability of her illness and finally the decision not to return to work:

> I'm aware of the demise of my health, again the pain coming, the breath-lessness coming back, the lack of energy again, so I just, you know, I just, the treatment will dictate, em, but that's also helped me decide I'm not going back to work, em, where before I was still thinking I could go to what I thought, I, I use the term 'normal life', but I don't think there's, normal that as I knew, it doesn't exist anymore, just have to create a new normal life, if that makes sense where its, its not working and its just sort of being able to do housey things, life things, family things but I've no work. (69, lung cancer, interview 3, patient and partner)

> Colleagues' attitudes and actions were significant if she was to shift her employment position because they remembered her as a 'live-wire, fun person, very capable at work... people came to me for advice.' However, she perceived herself differently after her diagnosis: 'You know, you get back to work in some form and everybody thinks that's it but it's not, its 100% different from what it was before the chemo, because there's a lot of thing that are different and you know, I'll never quite be the same person.' (69, lung cancer, interview 2, patient and partner)

In some instances the return to work was interpreted by others as a signifier of a return to a pre-cancer self. As described in further detail in Chapter 7, however, cancer for some people resulted in a changed notion of self over the longer term.

The impact of cancer on partners' employment

Adopting a systemic approach to understanding cancer necessarily also focuses on the role of, and impact on, entire networks of people around the individual diagnosed with the disease.

Policy (as described in Chapter 1) acknowledges the role that partners play in a patient's care. However, how active partners can be in providing care and support is impacted upon by the partner's employer, for example in their willingness to give them time off work. Facilitating taking time off work to care varies from workplace to workplace and is an area of negotiation because policy and procedures are not always in place or clearly understood. Some partners had the support of their employer or line manager. One partner was able to negotiate with his line manager time off work, which was a month in the first instance but was extended to two and a half months so that he could support the his partner during treatment. Others perceived that they would have to take annual leave in order to support the patient: 'I've got holiday that I can take so I'll just use up the holidays. I don't know how it goes, if you can take time off for partner's illness. I haven't looked into it. But I've got enough holidays to take to run you up and down [to the hospital]' (02, colorectal cancer, interview 1, patient and partner). Lack of clarity surrounding whether or not carers are entitled to paid leave to play a caring role is reiterated in the following quotation. The partner juggled work to support his partner during chemotherapy by using his annual leave entitlement until it ran out. At this point he was informed that he did not need to use his annual leave in order to do this:

> We basically just had to get ourselves a new routine going, based around the chemo sessions, so I had a lot of holiday left over from last year so basically I, where we did was every Friday, the chemo sessions were on a Friday, so I'd take the Friday off and then the week after that, when she was really feeling bad, I took the Friday and the Monday, so that used up all my holidays and I said after that I said 'right I'm just going to, I'm not going to take this as holiday, I've used up all my last year's holiday.' The work were very good then, they said 'yeah to be honest I mean you shouldn't have taken those as holiday', you know, fine. So I was able, you know to juggle the work round it. (12, breast cancer, interview 2, partner only)

Participants echoed the benefits of employer support but cautioned this with concern over whether the level of long-term support would match up to early expectations: 'I was working long hours, anyway … so they've had their money's worth out of me, but em, I think that … they are supportive … I think well, we'll find out how supportive they are, depending on what happens next' (12, breast cancer, interview 2, partner only).

Family members of patients contemplate giving up work altogether to care for their relative. A daughter explained that she had considered giving up work at some point if it was required of her: 'We don't know what to expect. I mean I might have to give up my work to look after Mum … when it come to caring for relatives and emergencies we [the family] all sort of pull together' (06, colorectal cancer, interview 1, patient and partner). Several partners shared experiences of how the cancer had impacted upon their own ability to engage in work. One partner explained that he no longer had the physical or mental energy in the workplace to help others:

> I would have been really been worried about things em or, or tried to, or maybe over-compensated to try and help them, where I say now, I just, I cannot do it because I've not got the physical energy, but I also don't want to use the mental energy because I need the phys, you know the mental energy for myself, so I've become a little bit more selfish in that respect.
> (69, lung cancer, interview 1, patient and partner)

Further, returning to a daily work routine proved difficult, as partners struggled to deal with being absent from home:

> He [partner] was saying 'You get back to work, you get back to work,' but I'm thinking, how can I go back and leave him on his own because he wouldn't even feed himself because he sleeps quite a lot just now, and he's no' got the energy … we've started going out for walks in the afternoon because it seems to make him feel better and he's not in pain when he's out walking. My mother stays down at … so we've been walking down there … he's been quite enjoying the wee walk. (17, colorectal cancer, interview 2, partner only)

Some partners took sick leave as a consequence of the diagnosis. This was because the impact of cancer was so detrimental to their own well-being that they were not able to work and they did not wish to leave their partner's side: 'That's me off work for a year, I was on full pay, now I'm on half pay … I cannot go back to my work and leave him you know' (17, colorectal cancer, interview 3, patient and partner). Working, at the same time as caring for someone with cancer, could be difficult, comprising of the need to keep work 'ticking over' while also diverting sufficient energy to care and support at home. One partner described this negotiation as beneficial: 'You don't have time to think about too much' (20, gynaecological cancer, interview 2, partner only).

Summary

As the introductory chapter describes, one use of the term 'whole system' is to emphasise relationships between different sectors and organisations that intersect with each individual's experience of cancer. At an elementary level, this chapter suggests that employment is a significant organisational system, which should be brought into the fold of joined-up cancer care to improve the lives of people affected by cancer.

Upon diagnosis, many people affected by cancer found difficulty adjusting to what was a new – and often traumatic – daily reality, and one which challenged daily living and transformed their relationship with their partner. For most people affected by cancer, diagnosis and treatment resulted in an overnight transformation of work from being a relatively well-managed element of their life to becoming a sub-system of a life now organised around cancer. Work plays a significant role for people who experience ill health. It is not only a key source, and often the only source, of income but provides a sense of purpose and structure in day-to-day lives. Ending employment, for example, is a life-cycle transition, which may be entered into prematurely, instigated by the cancer. Employment is often a key component of identity. Considering cancer in its broadest context must take into account the varied impacts on self and other that come about when there is a significant change to employment.

Chapter 7

Self and identity through cancer

This chapter focuses on the impact of cancer on identity. Identity is conceived of as something that is constantly in production, and is created through talk and inter-action. This is in contrast to concepts such as 'personality', which is considered a fixed and measurable sense of self. Academic definitions of identity are contested; sociologists draw on the idea that identity is 'the person we think we are. It is the self we know' (Christiansen, 1999: 548). For psychologically minded readers, ideas of *knowing* self calls into question elements of self that are unknown and remain outside of our conscious awareness (Cutcliffe, 2003). Thus, identity may go beyond what we know of ourselves and include what others know of us and what remains blocked from awareness.

This chapter explores identity which is apparent through people's accounts of illness, and draws on the idea that people's sense of self changes when cancer comes into their life. The appearance of cancer may privilege questions that have hitherto been pushed aside, to do with ontology and existentialism; that is reflections on being and existence. Existential concerns have been documented in cancer research for some time, for example Weisman and Worden's (1976) prospective study of 120 newly diagnosed people with cancer. Nursing research has adopted an overwhelm-ingly phenomenological stance to research, resulting in a pool of studies reporting existential concerns (e.g. Halldórsdóttir and Hamrin, 1996). In a position paper, Lee (2008) describes this as a hunt for meaning related to the still prevalent association between cancer and death.

Social scientists argue that illnesses with long-term consequences such as cancer, may trouble taken-for-granted assumptions about one's body and place in the world. This has been described as a 'loss of self' (Charmaz, 1983) or a disruption to a sense of self, generating a discontinuity from their former self to their post-cancer self. This has been explored in the medical sociology literature as biographical disruption (Bury, 1982), a theory which describes and explains reactions to chronic illnesses and has been explored in relation to cancer care (Cayless *et al.*, 2009; Hubbard *et al.*, 2009a). This connects with systemic theory, which argues that changes to identity can come about through first-order or second-order changes. First-order changes are those that are integrated into current patterns, or logical extensions thereof, whereas second-order changes are more fundamental presenting a discontinuity between past and present: 'second-order change has to do with altering aspects of one's world view and the basic rules that go with them' (Rolland, 1994:25). Thus biographical disruption and second-order changes in identity typify large shifts in a person's sense of self following exposure to a life-threatening illness.

A number of factors will mediate the impact and order of change of cancer on a person's identity. The nature of the cancer and its place in expected life cycles (for example a family legacy/expectation of cancer, which is discussed in Chapter 9) will play a role in the extent to which identity changes occur. For example, an abrupt diagnosis of cancer without previous symptoms or family history will potentially lead to more disruption and second-order changes. A second factor is related to social context and the idea that identities are social constructs that come about through interactions with others. Thus, how a person conveys an impact on their identity will be developed as a consequence of them as a social being, and as formulated in interactions with others. For both factors, the key component is to observe that identity construction occurs as a function of the intersection between the person with the disease and their social context.

Identity is a critical component of considering cancer in its widest contexts and systems. As Barber (2002: 2) suggests 'our sense of self is embedded in wider cultural narratives'. How cancer impacts on people's sense of self must become part of how people working in cancer care come to understand its widest influences. Without an appreciation of how people's sense of self may be altered, care will necessarily remain partial, privileging the physical understanding of cancer over a relational one.

KEY ISSUES

- Identities were clearly articulated as something that were formed and performed in relationship with other people.
- For some people cancer was disruptive to their sense of self, challenging them to think about who they were before cancer came into their lives and their new ideas about health, the future and relationships with others.
- Participants worked hard at maintaining a non-cancer identity by constructing themselves as having a linear and clear sense of self from past to present and into the future.
- People often asked themselves existential and ontological questions, reflecting a deeper reflection on identity and how cancer had unsettled their sense of place in the world.
- Sense of self was closely linked with the physical experience of cancer, with colostomy bags and fears of incontinence impacting upon how people viewed themselves and worried that others would view them.

- The notion of carer was called forth by many participants. Some people adopted this as a suitable new component of their identity, whereas others contested its relevance because they perceived it to be incompatible with their existing understanding of their relationship with their partner. This ambivalence to integrating 'carer' into people's identities is mirrored in the general care literature.

Impact of cancer on identity

Many people spoke directly about the impact that cancer had on their sense of self and who they are. Some expressed an idea of being 'obsessed' with it, with cancer rarely off their minds. Others indicated that the impact of cancer had been positive, in that they no longer worried as much about small concerns and adopted a *carpe diem* attitude, others indicated that they had made changes to their social lives to accommodate the cancer, which had resulted in feeling like a different person. The quotations below reflect the range and prevalence of such changes to self and identity. For example: 'You try not to say it to your wife and tempers start to fray. I'm normally quite a calm guy but now I'm on a short fuse all the time. It's just *bang*' (15, colorectal cancer, interview 1, patient only). For some people cancer had prompted a less positive outlook from their former selves:

> *Interviewer:* Has having cancer and the treatment, has that had any impact on your future plans. Do you think differently about the future now than you did before you were diagnosed?
> *Patient:* I'm a bit more pessimistic. Because, as you take options away, you've got less, that bit less to look forward to, right. In an ideal world I'd say look 'I'm not right.' (36, lung cancer, interview 2, patient only)

Thus a poor prognosis associated with this man's lung cancer diagnosis had led him to have to re-evaluate his life goals as 'options are taken away' and there is less of a future for them. This represents a disruption to the life cycle, re-evaluating an expected lengthy period of retirement and ageing and achieving goals and instead adapting to, and integrating, cancer. A further patient with lung cancer reflected on his diagnosis and was clear about how this had negatively impacted on his sense of well-being and thoughts about the future:

> *Interviewer:* Has it altered your outlook on life having a diagnosis?
> *Patient:* Yes, truthfully I wouldn't want anyone to know it, what's it all for? I'm feeling slightly depressed with it all.
> *Interviewer:* Yes. Has it made you reflect on life?
> *Patient:* Well I turn round and say, 'well, I'm seventy-two years old.' In my day when men retired at sixty-five years old they were dead by sixty-

seven, all related to industry, whether coalmen or whatever and I look at that point and say 'well I've got a good and reasonable life out of it.' I didn't want to change my ... way of life. I've just got to get used to it. And the biggest upheaval is I'm not going to get across to Spain when all this is going on. (46, lung cancer, interview 1, patient and partner)

For some people, cancer had prompted positive changes for themselves and their sense of place in the world. For the following speaker and many others in this study, the onset of cancer had begun for them a process of deciding to prioritise themselves rather than others from this point forward:

Patient: It's given me a different perspective, because when I hear that I'd been diagnosed, oh my Lord, I just thought, the bottom just fell out of my world. But now I know that, especially meeting other women who have go through it yes, it's a very, it can be a life changing this but, in a good way as well it's helped me review my whole life situation.

Interviewer: So you think having cancer has changed the way that you think about, or had an impact on the way you think about the future?

Patient: Yes, definitely.

Interviewer: Tell me a bit about that.

Patient: I'm not as scared as I was. It sounds weird I know, but I'm not scared as I was of a lot of things in the future now and, I'm thinking, I'm more prepared to take a few things that I didn't do before. I'm thinking 'right I'm going to do them now', I'm going to do anything drastic with my life you know big major changes. And I know another thing is I'm not going to, I'm going to concentrate more on my own life that I did before because a lot of my time was spent thinking about others and being there for others and I am thinking now, I'll be there for myself, that's what I am going to do in future, I'm going to turn wee bit selfish, as they say, and start thinking about my own life and what I want to do with it. (09, gynaecological cancer, interview 2, patient only)

Some participants explicitly reflected on the magnitude of change to their self, and connect this specifically with it being a *cancer* diagnosis:

It's changed, I think it's changed me as a person, I mean I think I'm, I think I'm more, I mean before I would have, I was pretty much, I wouldn't speak about problems, you know so, I mean if I, if I had any other illness apart from cancer I didn't think I would have spoke about it, but it's changed me, I feel now that I can be open eh, I really didn't give a damn, I mean at the end of the day you get folk moaning in the work about silly things, and you think pheeww! (28, colorectal cancer, interview 2, patient and partner)

For some participants the shift in how they viewed themselves was on a smaller scale. The following participant offered reflections on the small changes they had noticed in how they view the world: 'I'm not saying I'm emotionless, because I do throw the odd tear … I don't know whether I'm just looking at the world differently you know of the sun's shining, you can hear the birds…it's the stupid little things that you probably wouldn't have picked up on before' (50, interview 1, colorectal cancer, patient only).

Many respondents spoke of shock at hearing their diagnosis and taking time to fully process the meaning of this. A well-rehearsed psychological tradition provides an explanatory model for this delayed impact of cancer on identity. The theory suggests that protective (though potentially pathological) defence mechanisms manoeuver into the foreground, preventing the person from fully taking on board the diagnosis (Vos and de Haes, 2007). The following speaker highlights this, with the distancing between hearing the diagnosis and its impact on him described as 'surreal':

> But it was a surreal experience. It had nothing to do with me, I was sitting there taking this in, or not taking this in as it were, and it was going over me and when we came back home, the same kind of thing and it is still going on like that. I feel as if it is not me. And suddenly I will get nasty worries and thoughts in my mind about it and then it is not me. Surreal I think is the word to use. (03, colorectal cancer, interview 1; patient and partner)

Thus for some people the shift in sense of self was not immediate, but was a process, beginning at the point of diagnosis and evolving through treatment and into aftercare/follow-up. Some family members reflected on how cancer had impacted upon the person with the diagnosis, and drew on related notions such as denial as a way of trying to understand how cancer had been internalised.

> He did say to CNS 'I'm not in denial, am I? That you know I'm, I'm just very positive'. And people are saying to me that I'm very positive, and. That's how I, that's how he is, em, so we don't go about, eh, we don't talk about it. It's not that it's a subject not to be spoken about, you know it's not that. If I, if I said to him, 'em I think it might be good if you and I could meet with CNS, cos I do feel that I am more anxious than you, how do you feel about that?' He would, he would. He's very busy at work, but he would possibly say yes, or for me to go. I hadn't really thought … I think I was helping him by not demand, or not wanting to see CNS, but I can see that I'm quite an important part in this as well [laughs a little here]. (07, prostate cancer, interview 1, partner only)

A shift in thinking about one's self that was common, in people's accounts of their experience in the first year following diagnosis, was an awareness of one's own mortality. A diagnosis of a life-threatening illness, such as cancer, compels the individual to face hitherto avoided questions about death and dying. As discussed further in Chapter 9, and articulated by the following speaker, cancer in particular is perceived as a death sentence: 'The minute people mentioned the word cancer, eh, it's still a death sentence for, even though it isn't for many today, eh, but it's still at the minute a death sentence' (48, lung cancer, interview 1, patient only). Thus, people with cancer are faced with the prospect their own death, which they had not contemplated in the same way or to the same extent before: 'Yeah, when you don't know whether, you really, I'm saying "Am I going to live or am I going to die" and you've never thought of your own death. I, I never thought of my own death until then' (42, gynaecological cancer, interview 3, patient only).

People living with and beyond cancer had a changed view of living. Death, or rather the inevitability of death, now became a part of how they thought about their life and of themselves. The following speaker describes her situation as being in 'limbo' – between life and death. Although, ontologically speaking, all of us are between life and death, those living with cancer may feel in a different place because the prospect of death is much more apparent:

> It's limbo, isn't it. You know, I mean I've got my family saying to me 'Well after this mum, we'll go on holiday.' And 'After this mum, we'll do so and so.' And I'm thinking 'Oh yes that's lovely.' And then, and then something in the back of my mind is coming and saying 'Oh, but is it gonna work? Oh, but how many places is it?' You know. You're giving them false hope as well as yourself. And you kind of, you come back into, like a reality world. You like em to take you out of that and say 'We're gonna do this and we're gonna do that Mum'. Or 'Mum, as soon as you're well, we'll take you away on holiday'. You know what I mean. And I'm thinking to myself then, when they're having a cuppa or having the dinner 'Ah, but am I gonna be here then?' You know there's that … it's a death sentence hanging over you. And no matter how good a support group you've got, no matter how good your family is, that's still there. (65, gynaecological cancer, interview 1, patient only)

For some people, the onset of cancer had not 'added' something to their sense of self (such as the notions expressed above about worrying less about small things), but had troubled something which they viewed as a core component of their former self. For some this was epitomised in their changed view of their sense of overall well-being and fitness. For people who identified themselves as fit and healthy, cancer forced a reflection upon this. For many participants, both patients and family members, the presence of cancer in their lives had led them to a position where they were less confident of upholding a non-sick identity in the future.

> I don't think I'll ever go back to being, I don't, what, what I would ideally like is go back to blissful ignorance, so that when you've got something sore you didn't go up and go … 'oh I've' … like I mean I had a pain in my leg and I'm like every time you do it you think 'oh, is it cancer?' (70, breast cancer, individual interview, interview 2, patient only)

> You think well it really can't happen to me, I'm too fit. I climb hills, swim and I cycle … you name it, play golf. And then it suddenly hits you, 'gosh there is something seriously wrong here'. (15, colorectal cancer, interview 1, patient only)

This speaker, although building a sense of change to self through reflection on how this relates to his fitness levels, also manages a process of distancing himself from this realisation of the impact of cancer. His construction of 'something seriously wrong here' serves to distance the speaker from himself; that is, the use of 'here' rather than 'with me' enables a continued detachment between cancer and self. There is perhaps therefore some ambivalence toward a full integration of cancer into identity.

For other people, the impact of cancer on identity came and went as cancer entered and left their conscious awareness. Where it did stay in people's mind, there was a struggle to relate to cancer in a positive way, connecting cancer with victim-hood and weakness:

> You see them with the no hair and the no eyebrows and you think 'victim', and I didn't want to be classed as a 'victim', I didn't want people looking at me and giving me sympathy, 'cause I've got an illness. (28, colorectal cancer, interview 1, patient and partner)

> It really is sinking in, sometimes it hits me that it happened, other times I just, I don't forget about it but its always you know in the back of my mind and I just think, its not until someone says 'how are you feeling?' And wham [clicks fingers] it hits me again and I think I've got cancer and then I'll get scared but as I say, then I speak to other people around, that actually has it or have been through it themselves and that makes me feel, right I'm gonna be okay. (09, gynaecological cancer, interview 3, patient only)

Thus, for some people, the impact of the cancer on their identity was shifting not just between different phases of the illness trajectory, but on moment by moment basis as it entered and then left people's conscious awareness. For the woman above, this was triggered by conversations and interactions with other people. Identity is arguably always a social production. It can be seen most forcefully in instances such as those described by Patient 9. Exploring family relationships and cancer illustrated how many participants had told only a limited number of people about their cancer, so that they would not be perceived differently by others. For example, a man affected by lung cancer expressed a similar sentiment, indicating that he had yet to tell his daughter of his palliative diagnosis: 'Ignorance is bliss […]. But there's no way, I didn't bring her into the world to make her unhappy, so there is no way I am going to give her news' (36, lung cancer, interview 2, patient and partner).

Some participants were clear in the first interview that cancer had made no impact on their identity and it didn't appear to have a dominant role in their life: 'I don't think about it ... now and again "oh I've got cancer" but no' (50, colorectal cancer, interview 1, patient only). However, the notion of shifting and developing identities is brought to the fore when this same speaker reflects again on her experience. When interviewed for a second time five months later she reported an adjusted opinion in how much cancer was on her mind, but still framed this in the context of managing who knows about her palliative diagnosis. This was employed as a core strategy in enabling her to have control of how she is perceived by others:

> My immediate family knows that it's inoperable. My boss knows it's inoperable, but in general like, my friends and that they don't know. And I think it's more, well I don't want them to know to be honest with you 'cause I don't want people feeling sorry for me, and I think it's one of those things that, it's okay knowing that you have it, but when you have to come and say it to someone getting those words out you're like ... you know you're telling someone that, well you're going to die, you know, so em, basically only the immediate family know [...] I had to em, I had to enrol the children for their after school club em, last week and I thought I've got to tell this woman, 'cause you know she's going to be looking after my children. My children's behaviour is affected in any way then it's best that she knows what my situation is [...] I feel that if, if people know that then I could suddenly become the focus of attention and I, I, I'm not, I'm one of these people that would rather just be ... I prefer to be in the background. (50, colorectal cancer, interview 2, patient only)

The prospective method of this study, following people for a year after diagnosis, allowed for these changes in perspective to be identified and described. The speaker explicitly marks at the end of this second account how she perceives that one core element of her self has remained unchanged: that of preferring to be in the background, while she manages her cancer identity in relation to the staff at her children's after school club.

People's accounts indicated that professionals rarely held a very accurate understanding about the major impact that cancer and its treatment had had on them. The following speaker reflects a commonly expressed anguish about finishing treatment and the impact that this has on people's sense of self in relation to their cancer and the world:

> And then, the very last day of radiotherapy, sort of going up to the hospital that week, I spoke to one of the nurses and I says - well, you know 'Friday's my last day. Em, do I see a doctor or, or what happens?' 'You come in, have your radiotherapy and go home – and get on with your life' ... It's like you go away ... that's it. 'We've sorted you, go away'. That's, that's exactly how ... it was actually quite a weird experience the last day, going

up there, because it was like, well, you're on that roller coaster. (08, breast cancer, interview 2, patient only)

Thus, for many participants the idea that after a final treatment one could 'go home and get on with life' is at odds for the individual whose life and identity has been focused around cancer for many months.

Maintaining a non-cancer identity

The research data show that some people worked hard at maintaining a non-cancer identity, wishing to guard against being considered primarily as someone with cancer. For these people there was limited sense of biographical disruption, or of second-order change, in their identity. Indeed, some participants managed to integrate the experience of illness into their lives and sense of self, in a way that contained the illness. For people diagnosed with lung cancer (and therefore in receipt of a likely palliative diagnosis), maintaining a non-cancer identity was a substantial project. One participant was clear that they did not want to be viewed solely through a cancer lens, whereby her every action and utterance would be interpreted as being about the disease:

> It's a saying that I said all the time, 'life's too short' ... I have to stop myself from saying that now, cause people relate it to me and cancer and I, it's something I said for years, so I have to stop saying that and I also have to stop saying 'its not life or death' type thing, because once again it always seems like I'm relating it to me. (69, lung cancer, interview 3, patient and partner)

The following quotation illustrates how pervasive a diagnosis of cancer is in how people relate to each other. The speaker connects a conversation with someone with her own diagnosis but also how the other person had experience of cancer through her mother:

> Oh yes, I got flowers from the church, and em, the lady, the lady who brought the flowers, I said to her, 'oh well it's just one oh those things, you've got to get on with life', oh she says, 'I'm glad you look at it in that way.' I felt like saying to her 'well which way would I look at it, do I get depressed and say, that I'm going to get worse, or what?' I don't think people need to do that ... I thought it was a funny thing to say really ... her mother, I think, died of cancer. (54, breast cancer, interview 2, patient only)

Offering and conducting joint interviews with participants allowed people to construct together an idea of how cancer had impacted upon them. The following excerpt comes from the context of the partner articulating, at least to begin with, that the cancer had made no change to their life at all; maintaining a non-cancer identity. This is delicately, although staunchly, contradicted by the patient, who offers a range of illustrations for how the partner's role in the household has changed:

> *Partner:* It hasn't changed my life, I worry a bit, it hasn't changed my life.
> *Interviewer:* Are you doing at bit more?
> *Patient:* A lot more.
> *Partner:* Am I really?
> *Patient:* Yes you are darling, you're doing a lot more.
> *Partner:* But I cut the grass anyway.
> *Patient:* You cut the grass, you bring in the coal, things like that okay. But you're even starting to hang out washing and make beds on your own, which is totally new.
> *Partner:* Oh well I suppose yeah.
> *Patient:* You're doing cooking every now and again which is when I can't stand too long. You've taken over all the washing up, I don't do any washing up now. I'm a lazy twerp. Dreadful. (40, gynaecological cancer, interview 2, patient and partner)

For this couple, the division of household labour is used as the site of construction of identity. For the patient, this is around ceasing to contribute as much, whereas the partner takes up the slack. Although gender is not explicitly marked out, the type of cancer makes it clear that the patient is female, and that the household chores are now often being undertaken by the man. The partner positions himself as unaware of the changes to their domestic arrangement, and the subsequent impact on him; a feature which is not lost on the patient who clearly positions herself as having become 'lazy'. Thus, for one person there is an idea that cancer has not shifted their identity, whereas for the partner this does not feel congruent.

Maintaining a non-cancer identity was often expressed in relation to other people. For some, it was associated with a need to keep information from another person, so that neither of them had to manage changes. The following speaker highlights that for him, this is a pattern they have had throughout their life; keeping cancer to himself and upholding a non-cancer identity was therefore part of a life-long identity project:

> I'm not really interested in talking to anybody about it, nope. There's nothing they can tell me that I don't feel … I know I've got to get a job done and that's all there is to it … there's no use people going out praying for me and make it better because it doesn't. The damage is done it's got to be repaired. So there's nobody that can put your mind at ease if you're worried about it even if people do talk to you and you worry about it all, you're still going to worry. I keep a lot from [partner] … I keep things to myself, I've always been like that, I don't tell her anything because I'll only hurt her … she'll only feel hurt so if I can avoid that then that's what I'll do. (16, colorectal cancer, interview 1, patient only)

For some participants, upholding a non-cancer identity appeared to be a product of a coping strategy, whereby other elements of life were prioritised. This was illustrated in a range of ways, and the following patient typifies an approach whereby cancer was barred from taking hold of her, an aim which her partner joined with:

> I was, I got incredibly busy, busy doing everything, cracking that whip. (laughter) Just in the house and everything you know. I wanted all the decorating done before I went in to hospital, you can see that that's not happened, you know all these things, I wanted it all done and now I sort of just em, I didn't sleep well, I kept thinking. … I'm not so bad now but beforehand, before the surgery, em, I was just kind of just distracting myself with everything […] I was quite grumpy and irritable and em, emotional a bit emotional and I think little things were irritating me and then they would seem like a big deal and [husband] would be looking at me as if to say 'well what's the big deal about that?' And then I'd burst into tears and say you know 'can't you understand why it is a big deal?' And he would kind of calm me down and em, sort of you know make me realise that you know I just had to get through it. (55, breast cancer, interview 1, patient and mother)

For people of working age, maintaining a non-cancer identity was balanced with the need to remain in employment. One participant was actively seeking work and described the need to conceal her health status, feeling that the sick role identity would be one which would clearly mitigate her finding a job:

> *Patient:* I was quite worried actually when I phoned up because when I'd gone for my interview, I obviously hadn't mentioned anything about having cancer, I don't really think an interview is a sort of ideal place to go up and say, and at that point I mean I was, I've, I've always been pretty well through the whole thing anyway, and em, so I didn't, I didn't really think it was …
>
> *Interviewer:* Sorry to interrupt you but, it's just interesting 'cause I was just sitting there shaking my head [thinking] no, no interviews are probably not the best place and then I suddenly thought, well, why do I think, why, is it that you think that an interview … what do you think they would think, if you said you had cancer?
>
> *Patient:* I think they would probably just say 'no', because they don't, they don't know you and I think just on first impressions. I mean I go in there and that, they can see that I'm a capable person I can do it, but if I've got, if I went up and said that, even though they might think, that person looks really capable on paper, they might just think 'oh but she's got … what if she goes downhill?' (70, breast cancer, interview 2, patient only)

Why me?

Many people in this study had reflected on the perennial question: 'why me?' Charmaz (2004) suggests that the question is an identity one, as it poses a dilemma about the role of illness in the individual's life course, disruption to expected futures and notions of cause and effect. That is, puzzling over why cancer had happened to them prompted consideration of their place in the world.

People expressed a range of responses to the query about 'why me', with many expressing, for a variety of reasons, that this was not a pertinent question. For some, its irrelevancy was determined by an awareness that they had a hand in causing cancer through lifestyle behaviours or through hazardous work environments. Thus, although not wished for, cancer was not unexpected and therefore was not deemed to be as disruptive to identity:

> *Interviewer:* Have you, asked the 'why me' question in the sense that you
>   think it's related to the industry?
> *Patient:* Oh, I do believe that, yes. I do believe that. (46, lung cancer, interview 1,
>   patient and partner)

> I also know 'why me', because I asked for it a lot, by being a heavy smoker.
> (48, lung cancer, interview 1, patient only)

Genetics and heritability offered a similar range of responses, which invalidated the 'why me' question as pertinent to a change in their identity. This also positioned cancer as untroubling to a continuous sense of self: 'No, I'm doing what the, people have told me that it's mainly your genes, I've been told that it's in your genes, and that worries with my granddaughters, you know what I mean, that's the only thing I can think of' (65, gynaecological cancer, interview 2, patient and partner).

For some, there was a fatalism about cancer, so the 'why me' question was not deemed relevant. Many participants knew so many people with cancer that the question was not deemed relevant to them. Some people expressed that they had avoided any other serious illness or worrying life event so they didn't feel as though they had a right to pose the question. For these people, cancer had a limited impact on self, as it was already part of a wider cultural identity where cancer is an expected and normalised part of life. Others drew on Scottish truisms explaining why cancer had had limited impact on their sense of self from past to present. When asked if they had considered asking themselves 'why me?' one participant replied 'Why me? No. Well I haven't to be truthful, I haven't. Because I've always said "what's meant for you won't go by you"' (49, gynaecological cancer, interview 1, patient and partner).

Other people identified asking 'why me' with a spiral of negativity that was unhelpful and ultimately unfulfilling:

> Why you, why me, why us?, you know, I think we moved really quickly
>   on from that because I think we both knew that, if you get into that spiral

that it's a really, really quick downward spiral. (69, lung cancer, interview 1, individual interview)

Why me, what have I done to deserve this … yeah you do … Some days I don't think about it at all and then other days I sit and I cry my eyes out. Why is this all happening to me? (08, breast cancer, interview 2, patient only)

For these participants, asking existential questions of self was related to emotional reactions to the diagnosis. Shying away from asking 'why me' was then part of an overall strategy for managing this less valued part of themselves: the negative spiral of worry and depression.

Many expressed that it was a fruitless question, which held no satisfactory answer. They felt that it was as likely to happen to them as someone else. From this perspective, the impact of cancer on identity remains minimal, when it is shared by so many people in society: 'I looked at it and I thought, well, "why not me?" Why shouldn't it be me, compared to thousands of others? It's just it's one of these things' (34, prostate cancer, interview 3, patient only).

Asking 'why me' had led people to consider that if it hadn't happened to them, cancer might then have affected someone else. This kind of cosmic accounting, whereby one person's avoidance of disease led to someone else developing it was a worrying realisation for some. The following couple discuss their ideas about the selfishness of dwelling on why one individual over another should develop cancer:

> *Partner:* That's one expression that I do not like when I hear people saying why me? Because I feel if you say why me you want it to be somebody else. Why do you want somebody else to have it? We're all living in the same environment really, well the same world I mean you just think these things happen.
>
> *Patient:* It's happened, you know, so you've just got to accept it and make the best of it. (18, prostate cancer, interview 2, patient and partner)

Reflections also came in the context of discussions of a history of hard lives. One woman with breast cancer reported that she had already been through the mill with hospital treatment for mastitis, including a double mastectomy. To her, cancer was a further brutal blow:

But I think the first thing that everybody asks, when they finally come down to earth is, 'why me' you know. I've been through so much, I've lost both my breasts – not through cancer. I had very chronic mastitis 25 years ago and they kept … the lumps were really bad and they took me in twice and removed lumps and in the end the surgeon said 'the only answer is to take the breasts away and put implants in'. (13, breast cancer, interview 1, patient only)

For such individuals, though the cancer was unexpected, it came in the context of a series of health and life complications. The second-order change, or biographical disruption, is thereby mediated by previous experiences. The impact of cancer on identity evolved in the context of these other aspects to life.

For a minority of participants the 'why me' question was experienced as validating and useful. This was particularly the case for those who could identify no reason why, having lived virtuous lives, they should develop cancer.

> *Interviewer:* Have you asked the 'why me' question then?
>
> *Patient:* That was the first thing, why me, that was the first thing, as soon as the guy [doctor] went away and left me in the hospital, that was the first thing I asked, 'why me?' I didn't smoke, and I know smoking's not the thing, but you instantly tag smoking with cancer. Why me? I didn't smoke. I know guys out there that eh, I've had guys working for me that we've had to get rid of because they're abusing hard drugs, guys that are alcoholics. I've done nothing, I mean I've done nothing to get this. Why me? But, it's not an answer you get, you cannot get an answer to the questions it's just, and it is, I mean I suppose you probably find that's the question most people ask, is it? (28, colorectal cancer, interview 1, patient and partner)

Thus, identity was constructed in response to the oft asked question of 'why me' as a way of placing people in a social context, of hard lives, and responsibility or fate around cancer.

Physically embodied self

Identity and the body are closely connected, and particularly acute when thinking about the impact of cancer treatments on the body; whether this is the importance of the loss of a breast, the visibility of scars, or some other physical symbol of cancer. This is described in detail in Chapter 8; the current section explores the explicit work that people do in constructing their identity in relation to their physical experience of cancer. For many respondents, a change in sense of self was related to dramatic loss of weight prior to diagnosis or during treatment, however this was only one aspect of the way people viewed changes to their identity. The physical and psychological components of cancer colliding with each other was encapsulated clearly by one speaker: 'Funny thing is after telling me I had cancer I became ill and I became really ill' (36, lung cancer, interview 2, patient only). Respondents drew on very powerful imagery when describing the physical component to identity and how they maintained their public/social status. The following speaker likens the cancer, and his colostomy bag, to leprosy:

> Those that come [to visit] are very supportive and will use the word cancer. Others who don't sort of come, bow out, almost as if you are a leper. Added

to that the fact you have a colostomy which seems as if you are a further leper. Majority are alright. [laughs] We made no bones about it. There is no question when anybody asks us, they came to see us or speak to us we just told them exactly what the facts were. We have been very frank, tell the whole truth and nothing but the truth. (03, colorectal cancer, interview 1, patient and partner)

The notion of discredited and discreditable identities follows from Goffman's (1963) theorising around the social self and stigma, and fits well with people's embodied sense of self. Managing the impact of delicate toileting needs was a substantial component to people's identity work and their presentation of self in social contexts. Other participants reflected on how incontinence had impacted upon their identity beyond cancer, for example as being sporty:

Well the, the worst thing that bothers me if I was left incontinent, I think ... the rest I couldn't care less about ... you can imagine, you don't want to go about, walking about outside with a nappy on type thing ... I like going out on the golf course and let's face it, if you've got that and you did need, it means you've got to run into the trees or stuff like this, or you, you wet yourself when you're going round ... (34, prostate cancer, interview 1, patient only)

This speaker implies that the risk of incontinence intrudes upon his self-confidence, and possible stigmatisation leads to disruption in social situations. His worries about incontinence were sufficient to lead him to choose brachytherapy over surgery as having the least impact on his future quality of life.

One participant illustrates just how important the physical clues are, and frames this even in the light of his knowledge that he has a palliative diagnosis:

I did expect to lose a lot of hair, which em, so I was, I was built up, I mean that was the big thing, I wasn't, you know, it doesn't matter that you've got terminal cancer, you know I'm going to lose my hair ... everybody'll know, you know, that was, that was what I focused on because that was like something, I don't know maybe something petty or whatever, that I could just you know take away from that, but I only lost a little section along here. I went and got headbands. [and] I'm pre-warning people, 'I might look different 'cause I'm going to lose my hair', and I didn't lose, I mean I just lost a little section which I was able to hide, so again that was something positive, you know em ... (50, colorectal cancer, interview 2, patient only)

For some participants, their sense of identity was tightly wrapped up in ideas of their physical sense of self. The above speaker felt that their body gave away clues as to their health status, with hair loss, but felt reassured when little fell out. For another participant changed levels of fitness impacted upon identity:

> I used to be able to walk from here down to the bottom of the town, get
> a couple of groceries, walk back up again and not think anything of it. I
> worked for a furniture removal company, and I could run up and down
> stairs all day every day of the week. Take pianos, wardrobes, three piece
> suites you name it I could carry it. It was the easiest thing in the world.
> Now, it makes me sometimes feel like crying.

He goes on to say:

> I've changed out of all recognition. Especially the weight loss. I don't mind
> that so much. I'll tell you for why. Because I know that it's not something
> that I've done. It's the cancer that's doing this, not me [...] it isn't my fault.
> You've a lot of trouble convincing people, you know what I mean, you don't
> want to eat. You don't want to eat, there's nowhere to put it, you're not
> interested in it. Where do I go now? (36, lung cancer, interview 1, patient only)

For this speaker, the cancer is clearly separated off as something that impacts upon
him as a separate entity (this is explored more in Chapter 8 on the physical aspects
of cancer). It is so tightly woven with his identity formation, however, that he works
hard to ensure that the interviewer sees his cancer as the active agent in changing his
life. In the first excerpt, the focus is on his identity as fit and physically able, which
leads to a disclosure of emotional strain; the second passage develops the notion of
responsibility, placing control beyond self and onto cancer.

Tattoos were mentioned as a new element to their physically embodied self by
several people who had received them to help guide radiotherapy. These tattoos were
considered tangible and permanent reminders of their illness. One woman interpreted her tattoos as a mark of cowardliness, reminding her of how she felt forced
into having radiotherapy: 'To me they're a badge of being a coward and when I look
in the mirror I don't like what I see, I don't like what I am, I thought I was a bit braver
than that, and I wasn't that day' (21, breast cancer, interview 3, patient only).

People were aware of managing their identity in different social settings, including
work. Presenting oneself as having had cancer is problematised in the work context,
for both new jobs (as noted above in the conversation about when to tell potential
new employers about a cancer diagnosis) and returning to employment:

> Going back to work is a slight concern because I think there'll be expec-
> tations of me, because people remember me as being this live wire, fun
> person, very capable at work, you know - I was. I could, I could do a lot of
> things, people came to me for advice and, it's just the way I am em, and
> I thought oh my goodness I'm going back, and just physically not being
> as strong, does change things, I mean I would run up and down stairs,
> along corridors, you know have ten things going on at the same time, and
> somehow managed, be absolutely shattered. (69, lung cancer, interview 2, patient
> and partner)

The sense of living in a different, cancer-prone body impacted upon people's sense of self as a healthy individual. One participant, quoted above already, illustrates with clarity a sentiment which was echoed in many of the interviews:

> I don't think I'll ever go back to being ... what I would ideally like is go back to blissful ignorance, so that when you've got something sore you didn't go up and go ... 'oh I've' ... like I mean I had a pain in my leg and I'm like, every time you do you think 'oh, is it cancer?' (70, breast cancer, interview 2, patient only)

Thus, the onset of cancer had impacted upon how this woman viewed herself in the present, but also how she was anticipating her identity as a healthy person into the future. Cancer had disrupted a sense of well-being over her remaining life course in a way that had been unanticipated.

Contesting the identity of carer

Health and social policy tends to construct cancer as a family matter only as far as considering the paired positions of 'unpaid carer' and 'patient'. In this study family members played a far more involved and critical role, which has been described in Chapter 3. Participants reflected on their role and the appropriateness of the label 'carer'. It was not an identity adopted by many people, which connects with much recent research in unpaid care, where the carer identity is troubled and resisted (Forbat, 2005). The concern with taking on a carer identity is that this is given a different status to that of 'partner' 'spouse' or 'friend'. Although carers are canonised for their role in upholding community care, it is an identity that can come at a relational cost. That is, by defining the relationship in terms of care, this precludes a range of other valued identities that in turn impacts upon how families affected by cancer will respond and relate to each other. This debate sets the scene, therefore, for arguing for a specialised focus on relationships in cancer care, rather than the traditional focus on caregiving as the organising principle for family research and interventions.

Interviewees found themselves grappling with how to explain their changing role within the family:

> *Partner:* I don't care, like a real carer.
> *Patient:* Yes you are you're here all the time. You're with me, I can't go shopping on my own.
> *Interviewer:* It's a funny word isn't it?
> *Partner:* I cared before so there's ...
> *Interviewer:* Carer, because we've had a talk about that as well. What we mean by carer because a lot of people think that by care they mean dressing, you know washing, the other things that a sort of nurse would

do, you know somebody that was far more with a physical disability or something. People understand that term carer. What I mean is that person closest to you that then does all these things, a sort of enhances the things that you did do before but you know becomes more.

Patient: Slightly more.

Partner: I suppose it's slightly more. (40, gynaecological cancer, interview 2, patient and partner)

One person with cancer described his resistance to ideas of carers and being cared for. Its implication, to him was a threat to his identity and a concern about ideas of dying: 'At the moment I don't, you know, when you talk about "care" and so on, and how about carers, and, and I don't really want carers, I mean I'm perfectly well able to, you know ... I think there's, that, you know that you don't really want to think people into the grave ...' (64, prostate cancer patient, interview 2, patient and partner).

For this man, the notion of being cared for was incompatible with his relationship, and indeed forced a pessimistic shadow on his future. Needing a carer was viewed as recognition that the person's prognosis was poor. Thus for one person to take on a carer identity it enforced a dying identity on the other person; a feature which has not been developed in the literature to date. Another participant, the wife of someone with cancer, commented on how adopting a carer identity signifies a change in role: 'Well, I am a wife, I don't see my role has changed any because [my husband] has developed cancer' (03, colorectal cancer, interview 1, partner only).

Thus the carer and spouse role are presented as so similar that the different title of carer seems unwarranted. The interviews showed that partners provided crucial support and encouragement throughout the experience of cancer, beginning long before a diagnosis is given. The meaning of carer was deemed incompatible with the existing relationship. Additionally, people associated the 'carer' position with increased severity of the disease. The idea of being, or having, a carer represented a shift in the seriousness of the cancer. Thus the rejection of carer as an appropriate label goes beyond semantics and into semiotics. Resistance to the label demonstrates the active identity work that people affected by cancer engaged in, taking on board both their relationship with the person with the disease and the expected/anticipated prognosis.

Summary

Identity is conceived of as something that has both elements of continuity and potential for change, as a response to altered context and experiences. This chapter explored the way that people describe the impact of cancer on their identity and sense of self. Disruption to a sense of self was evident in many people's accounts, with changes evident from past to present and projected identity into the future. The impact of cancer appears mediated by the life course stage at which people experience the disease, and related notions of the extent to which cancer had been expected.

Much of this chapter has explored the impact of cancer on the identity of the person diagnosed with the disease. For family members, identity changes and reflections rested on their connection with being named a 'carer'. Interpreting the more marginal talk from partners/family members leads to reflections on how despite the notion of cancer being a 'shared disease' (as described in Chapter 3), its impact in identity terms is constructed as firmly located with the patient. Whether this is a function of cancer truly only resulting in negotiating changed identity for the patient, or if this reflects the lack of socially available discourses for family members to draw upon, cannot be resolved with recourse to this data, and should remain a subject of further enquiry.

Chapter 8

Physical aspects of cancer care

It would be easy to sidestep a chapter on physical elements of cancer, viewing it as a distraction form this book's main venture of seeking to enrich the ways in which cancer is understood. Rather than focusing concretely on the symptoms of cancer and side-effects of treatment, this chapter situates the body and physical experience of cancer in people's interpersonal relationships, and relationship with the disease itself. The chapter, therefore, moves through the familiar terrain of symptoms and self-care but with continued reference to how these are experienced in the wider context of cancer.

Cancer is necessarily a physical experience, although at what point it becomes such varies dramatically from person to person. Some individuals reported no symptoms or signs prior to their diagnosis, whereas others reported years of worries based on physical changes they had noticed. Part of the cultural backdrop of cancer is awareness and uptake of certain screening programmes (breast cancer being a well-known one with a population-based approach to screening), with newer additions in Scotland for bowel cancer detection. This sets a context whereby physical changes are interpreted and acted upon.

The chapter describes the range of symptoms experienced in the lead up to diagnosis, followed by reflections on the wider context in which the physical presence of cancer is experienced, locating it with other comorbid conditions. Specific treatment-related side-effects are then discussed before describing the myriad of ways that people recruited problem-solving to address physical effects of cancer and treatment. The chapter finishes by exploring how people relate to cancer as a distinct physical phenomenon, stepping outside of the assumption that cancer and person are symbiotic and indivisible.

KEY ISSUES

- The physical aspect of cancer is a core focus of the medical care that people receive while in hospital and using community services. Despite this, a wide range of physical sequelae are reported by people affected by cancer.

- There was a great deal of variance regarding symptoms experienced prior to diagnosis, and people's levels of concerns about those physical changes.
- People experience cancer often alongside a host of other illnesses, which shape their reactions to the cancer diagnosis and subsequent treatment and prognosis.
- The range of systems drawn on by people affected by cancer includes a variety of complementary practitioners and self-care techniques. Thus cancer care moves away from a purely Western medical model and into domains of expert patient and complementary medicine.
- The concept of 'externalising' was adopted by some people as a way of distancing themselves from the cancer. Externalising creates a boundary that serves to separate 'self' from 'disease'.
- Physical side-effects and symptoms are managed through people's own self-care strategy, with a primary focus on lifestyle behavioural changes, such as diet and exercise.

Physical symptoms before diagnosis

Some people reported no symptoms or signs prior to their diagnosis, others re-interpreted physical changes that they had noted in a different light following diagnosis, indicating that, with hindsight, they had an idea that they were ill. Other participants reported years of worries based on physical changes they had noticed; in one case the person had experienced symptoms for five years before a cancer diagnosis was made.

People were aware of basic signs and symptoms associated with cancer, in particular the presence of breast lumps and changed bowel habits (notably rectal bleeding), whereas men diagnosed with prostate cancer most often noted frequent urination as a key symptom. People with lung cancer reported the greatest number of symptoms including breathlessness, coughing (including coughing-up blood), chest infections and weight loss.

For patients without overwhelming signs of illness prior to diagnosis, a range of explanations were used. Tiredness, which was reported by most people prior to their diagnosis, was usually explained as being related to the ageing process or stress at work: 'Well, you know, I think it's quite difficult because you can look back and you can conjure up things so I am not really sure. I have over the past few months been saying I am very, very tired; I have to cut back hours at work' (05, breast cancer, interview 1, patient).

Meanwhile changes in bowel habits were often interpreted with minimal concern for their implications: 'I thought I was constipated' (06, colorectal cancer, interview 1, patient only). Another participant stated 'I felt I was having problems with my, well there was diarrhoea … I felt uncomfortable anyway, I wasn't, I didn't think it would be anything more serious than that' (38, colorectal cancer, interview 1, patient and partner).

One man with prostate cancer had not interpreted physical changes as symptoms of disease, and positioned himself as someone who was fit, healthy and taking active part in do-it-yourself (DIY) activities. He was one of many people with prostate cancer who spoke of pain as a symptom leading up to diagnosis:

> I had no symptoms, I had a sore back, em, around Easter time last year. I was actually doing a bit of DIY at the time, and I think it was actually sore before that it was getting quite, really quite sore with the DIY, and [I] went to the doctor, and he said well actually I'm pretty fit, never had a day off work for about 15 years or more. (07, prostate cancer, interview 1, patient only)

For other people, although they recognised symptoms their significance was minimised:

> Well, I noticed a lump, a small lump, and I spent a few weeks wondering if it was my imagination, you know sort of comparing ribs and lumps and you know I had [husband] feel it and could he, did he notice it, no it felt like a rib. I spent quite a while trying to I think, probably convince myself it wasn't there. (55, breast cancer, interview 1 patient only)

Another patient, who had lung cancer, commented:

> Yes er, the first time I just felt a sort of sore back, a pain in the, shoulders there, and I went to the doctor and, well I had a few weeks before I went to the doctor. And I did go to the doctor and she said it was, it felt like a muscle spasm and I had it for a while. (52, lung cancer, interview 1, patient and partner)

For others, symptoms were experienced and interpreted in the midst of busy lives, including the Christmas period which slowed the speed at which screening was sought:

> And I sort of jokingly said 'Oh and of course I've got a breast lump here' and I keep thinking I must do something. [My friend] said, 'You haven't done anything about it yet?' So I said, 'Well no I haven't really.' Then it was Christmas and New Year and I thought well I'll wait till after all that and then the thing that kind of made me move and do something about it I was standing looking at my breasts in the mirror and I thought that I could tell, I thought I could see a dimple. (55, breast cancer, interview 1, patient only)

Thus the experience of symptoms was heavily contextualised by elements of participant's lives, including the work context, lengthy periods of well-being and holidays.

Treatment side-effects

Treatment for cancer is associated with a range of side-effects that can cause significant morbidity, and can be life threatening. The process of symptom assessment is
fraught with difficulties including poor patient recall, retrospective assessment by
clinicians and lack of appropriate, clinically relevant and patient-friendly symptom
assessment and management tools (Lacasse and Beck, 2007). In addition, there are
recognised differences between clinician and patient perceptions of the emotional
stresses and experience of distress during chemotherapy (Mulders *et al.*, 2008). As
treatment-related side-effects are subjective, self-report is regarded as the gold standard for symptom assessment (Fu *et al.*, 2004).

Most people receiving chemotherapy or radiotherapy had been forewarned by
clinical staff of the range of possible side-effects. Disentangling side-effects caused
by chemotherapy and radiotherapy was, however, tricky since many people reported
receiving both forms of treatment in close proximity. Multiple side-effects were
common across treatment modalities, and many people reported tiredness, nausea,
hair loss, loss of appetite, a metallic taste in the mouth, breathlessness, sleeping
problems, constipation and diarrhoea.

A smaller proportion, across all cancer types except breast cancer, also mentioned
suffering repeated fluctuations between constipation and diarrhoea; and this was
particularly distressing for some. Hair loss was reported mainly by those people
being treated with chemotherapy for breast, gynaecological or lung cancers, with
around half of people getting chemotherapy mentioning it as a problem, and just
under a half of them using a wig. Additionally, a sizeable proportion of those receiving radiotherapy suffered post-radiation skin reactions.

People described their symptoms often, not as purely physical phenomenon, but
in relation to their impact on everyday activities:

> *Partner:* I think your mood really dipped drastically after the chemo-
> therapy at times, till you were really, really down.
>
> *Patient:* It did after the third one [chemotherapy treatment]. I was really
> down.
>
> *Partner:* But I think your symptoms contributed to your mood dipping and
> sometimes you didn't want to continue with chemotherapy, did you?
>
> *Patient:* [Daughter] came up one day and I was crying, and I don't usually
> cry and get down in the dumps, and I said to [daughter], 'I'm not having
> any more [chemotherapy], I'm not going back again,' she went 'I just left
> you alone until you felt better' and then she went, 'are you having any
> more chemotherapy' and I went 'yes'. [It was] just the way I was feeling,
> it just made us feel so ill. (52, lung cancer; interview 2; patient and partner)

The following speaker mentions a range of side-effects, and chooses to focus on her increased difficulty in keeping warm and subsequent impact on her heating bill and finances:

> *Patient:* I do get bad reactions from it. All these seizures and that, well not seizures, spasms in my nose and my eyes and my throat, my hands go, my legs go.
>
> *Interviewer:* Yeah, you said on your questionnaire you'd lost your appetite and that it was making you a bit depressed?
>
> *Patient:* Yeah, I'm forcing myself, I have lost a bit, depressed isn't the word, some days I just go mad. I mean it's like banging your head against a brick wall, I've had no help whatsoever money wise, other than the bit that Cancer Macmillan give me. I mean all right, I'm glad the weather's changed because I was putting thirty, thirtyfive pounds a week in here out of my money, the money that I was getting from the … what-you-call-it … Incapacity, course the bills have had to go, I've people yelling of money off me left, right and centre. (06, colorectal cancer, interview 2, patient only)

Another interviewee discussed her experience of flushes of warmth, articulating her difficulty in understanding their aetiology:

> *Patient:* …em, and I started taking that eh, I think in June that was and em, sort of get hot flushes, I got hot flushes from quite soon afterwards, I wasn't sure whether 'cause it was nicer weather as well, you know, but it does tend to, I do tend to get them like within a few hours of, of taking a tablet, I tend to get like a really hot feeling em, and first of all it was trying to figure out when was the best time to take it, take it and things like that as well, you know because it's em, you hear about the side-effects and you're like oh, I wonder if I'll get any of them and then, so I wasn't sure and so I tried taking it in the morning, but sometimes as well it makes, occasionally just sort of like em, just sort of lack of concentration, I just feel a bit spaced out, so I'd rather take it in the evening when I don't really have to think quite so much, rather than doing it sort of, I know some people take it in the morning you know, but I think if I'm going to work and things like that I need, my brains get affected, so I need to kind of em, try … so I prefer taking it in the evenings em, but it, it for some, I just seem to get, I do get sort of hot flushes, it's not really, really annoying but it, it just …
>
> *Interviewer:* Something you notice.
>
> *Patient:* Yeah, 'cause I'm, I'm, I'm always a quite a cold person, I'm always cold, and like my heating used to be, I would only, I would only switch it off in July. (70, breast cancer, interview 2, patient only)

People often reported that side-effects were notable early in the treatment regime, often at the first cycle of chemotherapy. Although healthcare practitioners may not express surprise at this, the function of such a framing in people's talk is to implicitly call into question how such side-effects might get progressively worse as treatment continues. The following speaker illustrates this neatly with reference to two different kinds of side-effects:

> *Interviewer:* So tell me a bit more about the effects that chemotherapy has had on you? You said it's altered your metabolism so can you describe that?
>
> *Patient:* Well, I just feel it's altered the body metabolism. Like I'm noticing now that when I shave in the morning there's not the same amount of growth there. Right. And that's only the first cycle. The other thing I'm noticing is I get an itchy face and if I rub hard enough, an itchy face, I'm just about the break the skin and my skin has turned a form of transparency. Now this is all since the chemotherapy.

Later in the interview, he went on to say more:

> *Patient:* Well to be fair it affects people differently they told me. My doctor (GP), she asked me if I've had sore throats or if I've had thrush. I said 'no, I'm just on the first cycle.' But I believe this could happen. It could happen, it doesn't happen to everyone. Not everyone their hair falls out she said 'it all depends on yourself' and she says that that, she gave me a mouthwash. (46, lung cancer, interview 1, patient and partner)

Other people, by contrast felt that the side-effects were more marginal than they had been led to expect: 'It wasn't as bad as I thought. It wasn't, and I'll tell you for why. I imagined it would debilitate me to the degree. But everything was gradual as opposed to, right, hair loss' (36, lung cancer, interview 2, patient only). Some patients spoke of specific side-effects, such as changes in their sensory awareness. The following speaker succinctly summarises side-effects that she attributes to radiotherapy treatment. It is noteworthy that despite these being textbook chemotherapy side-effects, she clearly marks radiotherapy as their cause, indicating how she relates to different treatment modalities and their impacts upon her:

> The treatment, the radiotherapy, I think, kicked in afterwards, there was this weird smell and weird taste and weird things, when I look back at it now the changes my body went through, I didn't see it at the time but there are a lot of things that I realise now that, yes, my body did go through a few changes, my appetite did drastically changed, I didn't even look at tea and coffee, I couldn't touch it. It was only cold drinks I could have and fresh food, I couldn't, processed food was just disgusting I just couldn't look at it. As I say I had this continuous smell from when I got home, I kept thinking there was a smell through the home, Mum says well I haven't, 'cause my Mum is staying with some friends for a few days, she said I haven't been

here there's been no … But it was, I think the chemicals of the treatment coming out because there are several other people I have spoken to have had the same kind of treatment and they said yes that will happen. This taste in my mouth I think it's like a metallic taste. Now and again I do get this kind of weird taste coming back but it's not nearly as drastic as it was and there's this kind of nocuous feeling and I get very tired easily. (09, gynaecological cancer, interview 2, patient only)

This speaker recruits her mother into her account, in terms of clarifying that these sensory changes were not as a consequence of her home taking on a new odour. Additionally, by reflecting on how her taste has changed over time, she too is able to explain these differences with reference to the impact of cancer treatment. She offers her own account of why these short-term sensory changes have occurred, integrating them into her understanding of side-effects.

For others side-effects were framed as being potentially a long-term sequelae of ongoing treatment. The following speaker struggles with other people's reactions to the end of one type of treatment and the onset of years of taking tamoxifen. She also connects the side-effects with broader gendered concerns about how treatment has impacted upon her ability to become a mother:

I don't like people dismissing it as if it was nothing and I, some people just seem to … most people that I know of wouldn't, don't say that, but a few people I've spoken to, and they just, they're just like 'but, but you're over it now', you know what I mean and it's, it's like but I'm not over it now, 'cause I'm still having, I'm having to take the tamoxifen. I've, I've got to have rubbishy periods, that's what, something that's just started as well, like really, really heavy em, periods that I had this month, took, took me completely by surprise and em, and, and like I'm not allowed to have children for five years 'cause I'm taking this tablet and I mean, I might not have wanted to have children anyway, but I'm not allowed. (70, breast cancer, interview 2, patient only)

A further speaker picks up a similarly embodied line of thought, regarding the physical impact of treatment and how she considers this important in how she wishes other people to relate to her:

Interviewer: Has it made you feel different about your body, the surgery?

Patient: It, at … but I think beforehand it did, and, but I think since like, since I was with this guy and it, it kind of reassured me that I don't look that, that bad, sort of em, you know like body image wise … I mean for a while I just oh yuk nasty scar, but now I don't really bother about it too much, you know so em, but I just …

Interviewer: Would you go in a bikini in the summer and things like that?

> *Patient:* Would I? Eh, no I probably would because, because the way my
> surgeon's done it, he's done it so you can't actually see the scar and,
> and in some ways I kind of like people to know it's there as well [slight
> laugh] … in a weird, kind of sick way, I just like em, like when, when I
> was wait., when I was going for the radiotherapy and I would like, 'cause
> it always got really hot, so I can't wear things high up my neck em, so
> I would have like a T-shirt thing on so you could see this burnt red bit
> sticking out and I, people, you'd think people would kind of look at me
> and things like that, and it was like, I wanted to say 'this, this is … I'm
> here because, I'm at the hospital because I have to have treatment, I'm
> not just here for nothing … it, it was like look, look see what I've got.'
> (70, breast cancer, interview 2, patient only)

For this speaker, the scars and signs of treatment were a motif of her experience, that she actively wished people to take note of, and integrate into how they perceived her. Thus for some people the physical signifiers of cancer treatment held great importance for their sense of identity, an idea that was explored in greater detail in the previous chapter.

For other people, the opposite relationship with the physical impact of cancer was expressed. One couple drew on powerful discourses of death camps to express the extreme emotional reaction the patient experienced when witnessing other people receiving chemotherapy. She begins by framing her experience as one of not knowing what would occur when she received chemo herself:

> *Patient:* That hadn't been explained to me like flushing out veins and how
> long the chemo was actually going to take and whether I would feel bad
> good or indifferent whilst receiving it and none of that was explained
> which I thought might have helped a bit.
> *Partner:* Yeah and I've, visions of, I've seen people with chemotherapy and
> you just associate it with people who might have come out of Auschwitz
> you know what I mean?
> *Patient:* Yes, that's.
> *Partner:* It's not the norm, it's they're just the ones you notice, you don't
> notice other ones. (40, gynaecological cancer, interview 2, patient and partner)

For men treated for prostate cancer incontinence and impotence were expected, feared and at times experienced by participants in this study. One participant alluded to impotence, but made it clear he didn't wish to elaborate on his experience: 'I think that's self-explanatory [laughs]' (04, prostate cancer, interview 2, patient and partner). Whereas a second participant said a little more about the long-term impact of his symptoms on his sex life: 'I had problems with sex, I just more or less stopped sex 'cause when I had sex it was painful … Two or three years'(34, prostate cancer, interview 1, patient only).

Another man with prostate cancer clearly outlined all the challenging side-effects of treatment that he experienced:

> It did what they said it would do, Zap the cancer. But it damaged all my other organs as well. My bladder was, I can't go without a nappy. My bowels weren't right and I had one morning at two o'clock I was absolutely pouring with blood and with burst veins at the back, piles. And I can't, if I am needing the toilet I've to run and I meant I don't get, I wouldn't have time to go upstairs if I hadn't a nappy on. (30, prostate cancer, interview 1, patient and partner)

Intimacy and sex were mentioned by a number of participants in relation to the impact of treatment side-effects and their altered physical sense of self. The following participant reflects on episodes with her husband as they managed changing ideas about relational intimacy:

> There has been some sort of inhibition, I think on both sides as far as sleeping together and I think that comment made me feel really unattractive and unappealing and he also says 'you know I don't know how you feel with all, all this treatment you've been going on I, you know I don't want to seem like I'm pestering you if your feeling unwell,' and quite a sort of lack of communicating I think from that perspective. And when I heard that comment I think it made me think 'oh my God I'm so unattractive' and, you know sort of, and yet he always hugs me and he's very tactile and he was mortified, you know, I could just tell that he was mortified about that but he, he's quite open about speaking about things. (55, breast cancer, interview 2, patient only)

Side-effects in the context of relationships were an important way in which people make sense of their experiences, beyond intimate sexual experiences. The following quote illustrates the impact of physical appearance on mood, and how this is connected to the wider context of people's lives. The date and event this speaker refers to is her son's fortieth birthday party:

> I hate myself at the moment. I really hate going out because I look … oh my skin at the moment … my face – I'm coming out in spots and … y'know I don't like the way I look!! 'Cause I was hoping to be able to get my hair … a bit of colour in my hair before the twenty-seventh but I don't know 'cause it's only nine days before the party that I finish my chemo tablets 'cause as I said I have lost all here [indicating her hair] but I don't know if it would take a colour yet. (06, colorectal cancer, interview 2, patient only)

Thus side-effects were manifest in the traditional ways expected as a consequence of standard cancer treatments. They were expressed however, not in a dissociated manner, but with their meaning and relational implications central. The next section documents ways in which people managed these physical components of the impact of cancer.

Managing the physical effects of cancer and cancer treatments

Managing side-effects of treatment also led to increased distress and difficulties. One woman reported how her compromised white blood cell count led her to increased isolation as she tried to protect herself from germs. This alongside her extensive hearing loss, meant that she struggled maintaining contact with others. In the extract below she refers to the symptom questionnaire sent regularly by the research team to monitor frequency and severity of symptoms:

> I have written down here em, in your em, because you've mentioned the questionnaire, there's a bit with emotions em, and there could be a space eh, like em, for the person's own comments and in that I would say, I personally would have added the part about em, in my loneliness eh, being cut off, and although there's questions about that, the end result for me was more coping with boredom, so em, I mean there is a bit, there's a space for adding comments, but the boredom thing is the one thing I would em, because I've had to isolated myself. Most people will only really probably need to isolate their self for the week or ten days that there blood count and their infection risk is high, but for someone like me, it's isolating. (31, gynaecological cancer, interview 2, patient and partner)

Around half of all people with cancer stated that they had been given anti-emetic tablets to help stop vomiting, but it is probable that many more were prescribed them. To some, the mere sight of their medication made them feel nauseous: 'It was getting, it was getting to the stage where you were being, you were being physically sick looking at the tablets in the box' (28, colorectal cancer, interview 1, patient and partner). This couple had developed a self-care strategy that minimised this problem and allowed the man with cancer to go to work for a few hours. His wife (the partner) described their process: 'What we've done now is, he takes his [anti-emetic] tablets in the morning and then goes back to bed for a couple of hours, he's fine because he sleeps again and that settles his stomach and then he can go to work in the afternoon. So this is what we've found since being on the chemotherapy' (28, colorectal cancer, interview 1, patient and partner).

Other participants reported the difficulties in managing pain, both in the hospital setting and at home. Managing pain in hospital was expressed with particular strength, set against an expectation of what analgesia people had anticipated to be readily available:

> *Patient:* Oh I had, I had thought it was going to be sore, there was absolutely no doubt about it, I didn't maybe realise the healing process would take such a long time, em, and no I didn't, I thought that the, I thought that

the pain would, would be dealt with em, and I don't think it was dealt with as, as well as it could have been

Interviewer: Right, can you say why, why not in terms of the drugs that you were offered or … ?

Patient: Yeah, I think it was in terms of drugs I mean because to start with em, what's the main drug that they give you initially?

Partner: Paracetamol and ibuprofen.

Patient: No, the drug, the main drug.

Partner: Oh, morphine?

Patient: The morphine it was whipped away very, very quickly, wasn't it

… (05, breast cancer, interview 2, patient and partner)

The same speaker, later on in the interview offers a second example:

Yeah, well I mean, well yeah, I mean there was one night, I was quite annoyed but I mean I must say this was, this was night 11, so you know this was my eleventh night in the hospital, so I mean, I wasn't in such a poorly state it has to be said, but I mean it was 10 past midnight that I got out my bed and went round, looking for the staff because they'd said to me at 10.30 pm, eh, my last lot of medication should have been given at 10 o'clock, so they come round at 10 o'clock and they do the last load of medication; 10.30 pm one of the auxiliaries had come in and said 'they are doing the rounds with the medication it won't be much longer now,' and I mean prior to this em, I would be clock watching and if I thought they had gone too far over the time when I should have had my medication I was buzzing them to get it, em, but as I say by day 11 em, probably could go longer between periods of, of not having my medication but by 10 past midnight I got out my bed and went, went through in search of them and had said to them, you know 'am I not getting any medication tonight?' I was really annoyed, but em, they said that my file had gotten put on to the file of people that already had, had their medication, you know which I thought was just [pause], I thought it was *bad* [laughs], I thought they're obviously not paying much attention, I think initially you know when you, when you really are very poorly, you know the, that time, first few days after surgery I mean they are excellent and they are always, always, I mean they are paying attention but I think they just kind of get quite lax.

(05, breast cancer, interview 2, patient and partner)

For the above speaker, there was a critical disconnect between the experience of side-effects and the unavailability of healthcare staff to provide medical management. The speaker invokes an idea that patients who are acutely unwell receive high-quality care; however, once this initial stage had passed, patients are left to fend for themselves, despite still being inpatients.

There were several ways that people with cancer tried to give themselves the best chance of their treatment succeeding through adopting lifestyle changes. Key components to this included monitoring and modifying diet, resting and aiming to be more physically fit. Around a quarter had changed their diet, eating less or cutting out certain foods (indeed, one woman with breast cancer became vegan as a response to her cancer experience). Others focused on including new foods into their diet (one man described his quest to find pomegranate juice), consuming more fresh or organic produce or taking dietary supplements such as cod liver oil, glucosamine and royal jelly. Partners and family members had been recruited into supporting the person with cancer to make such changes: 'My wife's been very good, what, what I've been eating is, she checking up in, in, in the supermarkets and that, that's there's non-preservatives in them and so forth' (46, lung cancer, interview 2, patient and carer).

A couple of people with lung cancer had given up smoking since their diagnosis. For other people, clinicians had made mention of smoking, but recognised that giving up would be particularly difficult in the face of the multiple stressors that cancer brings:

> *Interviewer:* Have they said anything about you smoking?
>
> *Patient:* Not really. Dr E brought it up one day and she said 'I am not even going to ask you if you've stopped smoking because it's stupid to even ask you because you've got too much going on in your head. You've go too much stress', she said 'I will ask you to cut it down a bit but I wouldn't even try to get you to stop'. I had cut it down a bit for a while, but I'm as bad as ever again. (45, lung cancer, interview 2, patient only)

Other people sought wider help with managing the symptoms and side-effects associated with cancer and treatment. Complementary medicines and treatments were used by a number of participants underlining the need to consider a broad range of practitioners in providing support to people affected by cancer. The opening utterance constructs also a difference between being healthy and unhealthy – despite the 'healthy' twin's own bowel troubles:

> My twin sister is, she's the healthy one … she's got bowel problems, em, so, so she, she goes to see this acupuncturist and she swears by him and her son's got eczema and he goes and he swears by him and they sort of suggested that he might help build up my immune system which is what it's all about, so I went 'yep, fine, I'll try it' and you know, and when I was pregnant with my second daughter, my first pregnancy was awful, my recovery time afterwards was just, like you know, about four months to recover, but with my second daughter em, I went to see this woman in Edinburgh and she did cranial massage […] I went to see (the acupuncturist) yesterday and em, he sort of stuck the old pins in the legs and the things and you know, I don't know whether, it's just that my blood cells are coming back up again

anyway, or whether it's, you know maybe to do with but I'm prepared to sort of buy in and if it's going to help build up my immune system, I'll give it a go. (50, colorectal cancer, interview 1, patient only)

Another speaker talks about a range of alternative healing systems, prioritising Reiki as one of the most beneficial to her: 'Definitely the Reiki, I would … I would go back and do that again … It's absolutely wonderful' (05, breast cancer, interview 2, patient and partner).

The longitudinal nature of this study allowed us to demonstrate the progression of symptoms for some people over the course of their illness and the debilitating effect this had on their lives: 'Breathlessness really bad, don't like it at all. I walk so far, don't I? [addressing partner] And then I've got to stop. I can walk so far down the road to the bus stop over this small hill, there's no way, I've got to stop, I'm out of breath. I've got to get taxis everywhere' (63, lung cancer, interview 2, patient and partner). In the following interview, five months later, the interviewee tells of his worsening symptoms 'I coughed up some blood last week didn't I? Coughed up some blood. I says right, breathing really bad, exceptionally bad. I can't go out […] and I've got wheezing. Do you hear it? I can't get rid of this bloody wheezing in my throat'.

For patients with life-limiting cancer, worsening of symptoms led to a refocusing of their and their family's priorities and often a change in services:

> Being [at the hospice] also happens to be very close to where my family live, a lot of my family and my dad em, I thought who doesn't drive, I'd probably feel quite 'safe' … I'm sure he would, sadly he'd want to come and see me, he could come and see me, without too much trauma, having to get all the way through to the west here, because [my partner] and everybody through here drives. So I suddenly thought it'd make it easier and I wouldn't be worrying about him em, which is important em, so and the staff there, you know they, they're, well they're excellent, you know that's what they're trained for and a lot of them have been through cancer and such like, so they understand. (63, lung cancer, interview 3, patient and partner)

This awareness of limited prognosis facilitated preparation for the future and impending death and for this individual the need to consider her family at this time.

Comorbidities: the relationship of cancer with other illnesses

A significant proportion of the cohort of this study had pre-existing conditions, which contextualised their reactions to cancer. The sub-title indicates not that there is a causal relationship between two or more conditions, but that they are understood and interpreted in the light of each other.

For some individuals, cancer was added to a long list of other conditions that they were living with and took on no particular significance. The onset of cancer was not therefore considered to be a disruption to their physical being or to their sense of self. For some individuals, these other health problems were clearly considered more pressing than the cancer. The following speaker has organ failure, which may lead to him having a far poorer prognosis than from his prostate cancer: 'I've actually I've been suffering from chronic kidney failure at the moment. And I've sort of taken a sort of turn, eh for the worse in the last, shall we say, couple of weeks! So I'm *now* perhaps going onto dialysis! In fact I'm getting lined up for dialysis some time in May, or or *preparation*, sorry preparation for dialysis' (43, prostate cancer, interview 1, patient and partner). One interviewee had a long history of complex health problems including autoimmune disease (Sjogren's syndrome), extensive hearing loss (since the age of 26) and tuberculosis (TB). She describes how these impacted upon her experience of cancer: 'The worst isolation is boredom, at home. Because of my blood and em, my former TB, maybe reactivating my Sjogren's syndrome things em, I could, I have to keep away from where there's people and because my blood is never [right]' (31, gynaecological cancer, interview 2, patient and partner). This participant also explains that it is these underlying conditions, in addition to the side-effects of treatment, that are of concern to her. She identifies that it can be hard to disentangle where symptoms stem from:

> *Patient:* [I've had] no nausea or vomiting afterwards, em, nothing, nothing, nothing to report other than the fatigue. A little problem with sleeping, but that's also Sjogren's syndrome em, a little trouble with my legs on carboplatin … eh, but em, it's difficult when they ask you in the [hospital name] eh, for the, for the past month, because so many of my things I had with Sjogren's syndrome anyway, so, I can never assess.
>
> *Interviewer:* It's hard to tell which is due to the chemotherapy and …
>
> *Patient:* That's right. I got through a couple of awkward phases with my legs
>
> *Partner:* Aye, when she's walking sometimes she tends to stagger a little bit left or right … she pretends she was going that way anyway! [laughing]
>
> *Patient:* And I've got to hold onto him if he stops to speak to somebody or em, I want to look at the nice car, you know the kind of thing [laughs]; uhh uhh, they're quite weak. (31, gynaecological cancer, interview 2, patient and partner)

Other participants had more common ailments that pre-dated the cancer diagnosis, and created a puzzling history in which people were uncertain how to attribute physical changes they had noted. The following couple jointly construct the complexity of disentangling symptoms:

> *Interviewer:* What sort of symptoms did you have?
>
> *Patient:* Just this pressure. It's like, it's like constant constipation, as if you want to go to the toilet and you sit and squeeze and squeeze like

toothpaste, and forget it, nothing happens. This is why I thought I had piles because I had forced it, but as it turned out it wasn't.

Interviewer: What about anything else? Did you feel tired?

Patient: Oh aye, felt tired.

Partner: Tired all the time really, definitely couldn't walk at all. Having to stop every few yards. In fact we didn't, I eventually went out for wee walks on my own.

Patient: I've got an arthritic hip as well, that doesn't help! [laugh]

Partner: That's the problem. [Patient 01] was blaming all this on his hip, but it may never have been that.

Patient: I think it was the pressure on a nerve somewhere inside that caused the pain down my leg.

Partner: In actual fact for all that time you were saying you couldn't walk, because he's got a steel pin in his ankle and he assumed it was causing arthritis in the hip, but I truly don't think that is the reason at all. So if we go by that, I would say it must be about a year, he's been unwell. (01, colorectal cancer, interview 1, patient and partner)

At other times, symptoms were interpreted by people as being indicators of other, as yet undiagnosed, illnesses. One woman told of how her two years of symptoms before being diagnosed with colorectal cancer had led her to consider a range of possible, and very worrying, diagnoses: 'But I mean sometimes you used to have to wait three weeks. But my head was scrambled as well. I thought I was getting Parkinson's or something like that senile dementia. It got to the stage that may be it is all in my head because I couldn't remember things' (06, colorectal cancer, interview 1, patient and daughter). Thus, the experience of the physical presence of cancer was mediated for many by coexisting conditions, and concerns about other diagnoses formed the context for responding to emerging symptoms.

Relating to cancer

A core component to understanding the physical sequelae of cancer is to consider people's relationship with the disease itself. The idea of externalisation is a useful way of conceptualising this, and has been integrated into systemic thinking over the past decade, and has taken a very powerful and somewhat new approach to thinking about illness. At its core, externalising takes an illness, or a behaviour, and locates it outside of the individual – so the problem is no longer located within the individual, but is considered external and self-determining.

This has been used to powerful effect by therapists working with families with a range of concerns, such as anorexia, aggression and attention-deficit hyperactivity disorder (Epstein, 2008). Therapists might approach externalising in a way that suggests that the problem has its own will and independence from the individual, asking 'when did depression come into your life?' 'when does depression get the better of you?' 'when do you manage to overpower depression?' This approach is powerful because it serves to separate the person from the 'problem'.

In a more subtle form the notion of externalising might be used in daily discourse in marking a difference from 'I am depressed' to 'I have depression'. For cancer, this notion of externalisation has particular salience. It marks cancer as something that is not only located as a physical blemish to the individual, but something which is also external to them and has a life of its own. Its independent life is created by the social context in which cancer is understood and related to. Externalising cancer has a salience that is readily identifiable, since cancer has its own physicality. It is not a leap of ontology, as it can be with anorexia or aggression, to recognise it as autonomous to the individual in which it is situated.

One couple illustrate this notion perfectly, reporting the speech of the doctor who informed them of what the surgical team had discovered:

> *Partner:* We told you about after the operation, 'well, she has cancer in the ovaries.'
> *Patient:* Has? That sounds as though you've left them in there [laughing].
> *Partner:* It's just the lack of the English words. Yes her ovaries are in a laboratory somewhere.
> *Patient:* They're in a little glass jar and they've got cancer [laughing].
> *Partner:* Yes. But the way it was put. (40, gynaecological cancer, interview 2, patient and partner)

For this couple, cancer was presented to them at diagnosis as something that was dissociated from the woman herself, to an extent, they underline this by reiterating that the ovaries are 'in a little glass jar' and *they* (not the woman) have 'got cancer'. Another participant extrapolates this idea of externalisation even further, nominating the cancer its own name and identity:

> When I had the operation I was told I needed it. I mean I named it ET – my tumour alien – being you see and even right the way down to going down for the operation I was laughing and joking, they said 'are you not scared?' and I said 'no I'm getting rid of ET!' They said 'what d'you mean ET?' I said 'my alien being inside me' I said 'it's gotta come out' I says 'what's the use of worrying?' (06, colorectal cancer, interview 2. patient only)

People often spoke of how their relationship with cancer had changed from previous understandings of it, through family members developing the disease. The following extract illustrates this shift was felt by both patient and partner, as they reflected on mutual friends who had experienced the disease:

Interviewer: You talked before about all the people that you know have cancer and some people, you know your fear of the cancer treatments in terms of the chemotherapy, now that you've had experiences of it and sort of lived it, has it had an impact on the way you think about what cancer is and what happens to people who have cancer?

Patient: My main idea of cancer was having nursed my mother through her terminal cancer and that did somewhat colour my outlook when I learnt that I had it [...] It used to be a death sentence. I don't believe it is.

Partner: Especially when two people have had it away back in the [unable to make out].

Patient: And then I thought of a friend whom I used to work with in London and she had cancer, ovarian cancer I'm sure it was ovarian. She survived well into old age.

Partner: She was in her eighties wasn't she?

Patient: So you know it balanced out. Eh, our friend in [location] died of cancer, but it wasn't diagnosed in time. But no I went into a thinking of yes you know it's not a death sentence I have a chance of survival. And I think you believed that as well didn't you?

Partner: Oh God yes. (40, gynaecological cancer, interview 2, patient and partner)

Another patient expressed how her relationship with cancer had changed, noting in particular how her view of it as a necessarily terminal illness had shifted dramatically:

Interviewer: Has having had cancer changed the way you think about cancer and what happens to people who have it?

Patient: Yes it has. I mean probably through my own, I don't know if the naivety or ignorance, before I was one of these type I thought, as soon as I heard I had cancer I thought that's going to be it you know. To some a definite death sentence to others, you know going through like on medication and this, that, the next thing for the rest of your life and now I understand that cancer is not something like that any more. A lot of types of cancers can be you can cure it, it is a curable thing and maybe within, hopefully within my life time we might see them all being cured. (09, gynaecological cancer, interview 2, patient only)

Summary

People experience a wide range of symptoms associated with both the cancer and with treatments. For many patients the first indication that there may be something wrong is a physical manifestation of disease such as a lump or changes to normal functioning. The physical consequences of cancer permeate the cancer experience for both the patient and their families. The impact of symptoms on people's lives is evident from the accounts illustrated above, as is the complex way individuals ascribe meaning to these symptoms. What is evident from this study is that much remains to be achieved in routine clinical care to assess symptoms more effectively and intervene appropriately.

In addition, consideration of the concept of externalising cancer may afford greater understanding for professionals in the way people affected by cancer make sense of their illness.

Chapter 9

The social contexts of cancer

The central tenet of this book is that cancer is not experienced by an individual in isolation. Much of the writing to this point has focused on the immediate interpersonal relationships that the newly diagnosed person with cancer is immersed in. This chapter broadens out, and includes a much wider sense of context. To paraphrase Bateson (1973), there is no meaning without context. That is, without knowing the situation in which a person is diagnosed with cancer, its meaning and implications will remain obfuscated. 'Contexts' is purposefully plural; it indicates the breadth of influences that impact upon cancer experiences and the articulation of cancer care.

Clinical teams in cancer care rarely have more than a narrow understanding of the wider contexts of the lives of the people they diagnose and treat. This was evident in the research interviews conducted during the course of this study. With large numbers of patients moving through clinics, this does not register as a surprise. Thus one of the aims of this chapter is to draw on the research interviews with people affected by cancer, to illustrate the complex contextual layers which inform and frame people's experiences of cancer, in a way that may be difficult to elicit in demanding everyday clinical practice.

KEY ISSUES

- How cancer is understood and experienced will be mediated by the contexts in which it occurs.
- Contextual layers are identified and discussed in relation to systemic theory known as CMM (the Coordinated Management of Meaning) as an explanatory framework for cancer care.
- Culture, religion, social environment, family beliefs and individual experience are all considered important contextual layers.
- People draw down from different contexts to make sense of and articulate their experiences of cancer.
- A full understanding of the impact of cancer on people's lives can be better reached when the complexities of different mediating contexts are highlighted and can be considered.

Excavating cancer contexts using systemic theories

This chapter draws on a theory developed and utilised within family therapy circles, known as CMM, or the Coordinated Management of Meaning (Cronen *et al.*, 1989). The theory draws attention to different interconnected levels of context, in which experiences are understood and interpreted.

At its core, CMM proposes that to understand meaning, one must understand context. An oft quoted illustration of this is the necessity of contextual information to create meaning around an act of killing. One context (war) may mean a legitimised death, whereas another context (domestic abuse) creates a meaning of unlawful murder. Thus, the same act in different contexts necessarily results in different meaning-making.

In terms of understanding cancer, important contexts include cultural, religious/spiritual belief systems and personal life stories. To organise these various ideas of context, CMM adopts a hierarchical system ordering the different components in increasing layers. It provides a platform for identifying (and thereafter working with) the different contexts that mediate people's experiences of cancer and cancer care. The hierarchy model forces attention to a broad range of systems that influence how cancer is experienced. For some people, the highest context might be one of religion, under which all others are subsumed; for others the medical discourse may be the highest level, subjugating other contexts, and thereby marginalising other meanings and interpretations. Montgomery (2004: 351) provides a useful summary of CMM: 'Social meaning is seen as organized in a hierarchy in which each level is understood within the context of a higher level, and is also the context for understanding the lower levels. The number, nature, and place of levels in the hierarchy are not predestined, and although they are drawn hierarchically, they are all equally important.'

Further, the highest context (the one organising all other interpretations and understandings) can shift. Thus, the positions within the hierarchy are not fixed; and the most dominant context can change (Cronen *et al.*, 1989).

Coordinated Management of Meaning has been proposed as a practical theory (Barge, 2004) and has been applied in related fields, such as dementia care, to illustrate the complexity of issues that mediate people's experiences of ill health (Forbat and Service, 2005). The model enables us to look at how meaning is created within social interaction. It refers to the multiple layers of context that influence interactions and meaning-making. In this chapter, CMM is therefore used to excavate the important social and cultural contexts in which cancer is experienced and illustrate how they mediate and feed into people's understandings of and responses to cancer.

Cultural mediations of cancer

Culture refers to a set of shared beliefs, attitudes and values that are held by a particular group: for this study, culture relates to the particular socio-historical space of early twenty-first century Scotland. It is elements of this culture that can be identified within the interviews and that shed light on how cancer is articulated and related to.

The study was undertaken at a time when the media is saturated with accounts of cancer (Johnston, 2005). During the time of the research, well-known people in the public eye were treated for cancer: Kylie Minogue, Diana Moran and Sheryl Crow, for example, were all diagnosed with breast cancer. The media reported dozens of biomedical studies that pointed toward more effective treatments, and work which indicated risk and protective factors. All these media representations of cancer contribute to the cultural milieu in which cancer is experienced and impacts upon people's understandings of the disease and relationship with it. Anecdotally, and in line with this high media profile, there is an understanding that speaking about cancer is now more socially acceptable than it was some fifty or even twenty years ago within UK culture. The following participant explains how she views the cultural shift in how people have related to cancer over time. She talks of a relative who had been diagnosed with a similar cancer some years ago:

> Aye, it was, there wasn't screening then, you see, she's been, she died in 1986 so that's twenty year ago you see and there wasn't as much, there maybe was screening then but, well we stayed in, she stayed in [town] maybe there was none, maybe they didn't come there, I don't remember, but, but you know, people are funny twenty years ago, cancer was a kinda taboo, you know, you didn't speak about it. (54, breast cancer, interview 2, patient only)

This speaker talks more about this idea:

> *Patient:* That is the scary bit. I mean I, I've got friends this year who are fifty-two and this is the first time that they've had mammograms ... and, like as I say, I'm only forty-seven and that is the, the, the scary part about it ...
>
> *Interviewer:* What do you think has changed?
>
> *Patient:* Well people talk about it and they, they just talk openly about it, cancer's another disease like other things and, it's just, it, it's talked about and discussed and ...
>
> *Interviewer:* Yeah, so what did, what was different before then that people didn't, you know that was making it taboo?
>
> *Patient:* Well there was such a, it was such a death, you know if you had cancer, you were going to die, there just, there was no hope ... (54, breast cancer, interview 2, patient only)

Thus people's understandings of the cultural context of cancer informed their views of the disease, viewing it as one that has reduced in its taboo, which can now be openly discussed without fear of immediately implying death. As the following speaker suggests, cancer and death have to some extent been de-coupled 'It used to be a death sentence. I don't believe it is' (40, gynaecological cancer, interview 2, patient and partner). This articulation of cancer as no longer being a 'death sentence' was common. In this next quotation the partner draws on clinical evidence to explain the cultural shift in the perception of cancer: 'There is such a, such a good percentage recovers from it, which is a good thing, I mean at one time of day it was, it was a death sentence' (09, gynaecological cancer, interview 1, partner only).

Yet cancer remains strongly associated with death. The following quotation suggests that cancer is simultaneously associated with living and dying; some people may live with and beyond cancer whereas others die from the disease. It is this contradiction that is contemplated by those who experience a life-threatening illness such as cancer: 'Normally if you get people who've got cancer they go downhill quite quickly and then I think me, for what I've been through it's demonstrated to them it's not a death sentence once you can bounce back from it, if you keep everything right and it depends on how you got it' (28, colorectal cancer, interview 3, patient and partner). This cultural shift whereby cancer is no longer perceived as a 'death sentence' is, therefore, not complete and all-pervasive and it does not serve to alleviate the fear of cancer. Thus, people may acknowledge that cancer is no longer a death sentence but still remain somewhat fearful. The following speaker describes her mixed emotions. She wishes to be optimistic but she is so very afraid:

> I feel part, yeah fear, depressed yeah, not too depths of despair or depression because as I said what I'm getting into my head is it's not necessarily a death sentence. It's something I'm going down to come back up again. Optimism as well, thinking oh it's …. Yeah anger, frustration. I've got mixed emotions going through. Thinking obviously you know 'why me?' and also when I'm looking through all the news and everything that I see all these people that have to go to hospital and have all these things and I think I look at them and think … now it's happening to me, my God. Now I can understand the trauma and the fear and the yeah and I think that was a very scary part of it. […] I thought that's bound to be … not panicking because I'm not at death's door. I don't feel I'm at death's door. I really feel perfectly healthy. (09, gynaecological cancer, interview 1, patient only)

Participants offered further views on cultural discourses of cancer and serious ill health. Cancer is constructed as a 'silent' disease which may stalk someone and strike when they are least expecting it. Several people with different cancers identified theirs as the 'silent' disease, which shows few symptoms before the disease has progressed substantially:

> They have no way of knowing how ovarian cancer starts, but I've been ill since I was eighteen, I have never ever said 'why me?' I, I really, really

have no time for anyone who says 'why me?' … But as for ovarian cancer I have no idea, they have no idea. The silent killer, it comes up on you, it can be coming up on you for a while. I, I would think every cancer, I look on cancer as 'an evil' because, it's so, it's in the night the thief in the night, and then suddenly you know 'he's' there. (31, gynaecological cancer, interview 2, patient and partner)

Partner: They say bowel cancer is the most researched cancer for, they know more about that bowel cancer, they know more about the bowel cancer, it's one of the more silent one as well, so people can have it and don't know that they …

Patient: That the big thing that everybody in the work as saying to me is that I'm lucky. (28, colorectal cancer, interview 1, patient and partner)

A further participant drew more widely on culturally available ways of understanding how sly cancer can be in hiding without significant symptoms. He begins by contextualising this understanding of key symptoms for lung cancer before offering an account of his friends' attempts to calm the worries he had prior to being diagnosed:

It's interesting, for all the breathlessness, em and the pain, and the tiredness which I had had, and I thought oh maybe there's a link there now, em, I still felt then OK as I do now, you know I didn't have any other effects, em, ill health, so I thought that was that, and I just didn't think any more and a couple of people at work that I'd spoke to said 'oh, don't worry, you know the painful things are not the serious things'. (69, lung cancer, interview 1, patient and partner)

Cancer, therefore, is understood as something that is more socially acceptable to speak of, yet still contains a sense of being an illness that may creep up on people. By constructing cancer as not always announcing itself immediately, people are able to manage the impact of the illness on their identity and account for how far the disease has progressed without it becoming known to them. This connects with the discussion on identity developed in Chapter 7.

The simultaneous characteristics of cancer as being something that can now be openly discussed and as being somewhat sneaky in its appearance in people's lives both inform how people relate to cancer. Running alongside this, is the notion of taboo, which although no longer casting its shadow across cancer as a whole, still plays a powerful role in discourses of blame and the presence of cancer in people's lives. This was particularly visible in talk around smoking.

Thus, a culturally available way of speaking of cancer in contemporary Scottish society is the place that tobacco occupies as a cause of disease. The ban on smoking in enclosed public spaces was introduced during the course of this three-year programme of research, and was thus in the news on a regular basis, reinforcing messages about the risks of smoking (Scottish Government, 2005). Personal responsibility for cancer (and blame) has become a prevalent way in which the disease is constructed, and is reinforced by public health messages around tobacco. The majority of speakers drew on ideas of tobacco and smoking as they expressed their views on their own cancer's aetiology and as a general risk factor, and accounted for their own ill health with reference to smoking. These features of the interviews indicate how pervasive smoking is as a culturally available way of explaining and talking about cancer. Accounts were often peppered with movements between recognising smoking as a risk factor, yet minimising its saliency in their particular circumstances. The following speakers were among several who discuss the aetiology of cancer in relation to asbestos:

> *Partner:* Dr F [consultant surgeon] put it down to your industrial career, didn't he? It's nothing to do with, you know when people are asking you?
>
> *Patient:* I was quite a heavy smoker in my younger days. I smoked a pipe and cigars.
>
> *Partner:* That wasn't the kind of cancer you had, it didn't come from smoking.
>
> *Patient:* It wasn't smoking related, no.
>
> *Partner:* It wasn't smoking related. It was, your in the jobs in industry you'd been in. Because there's still little flecks of asbestos. They showed us these floating in his lungs when we were looking at both the CT [computed tomography] and the X-rays. (44, lung cancer, interview 1, patient and partner)

Thus in the above extract, the speaker indicates that it was the consultant surgeon who identified the external cause of the cancer, enabling the couple to disregard the impact of smoking on the disease. A further example from another participant illustrates the delicacy with which smoking was managed between family members, as the person with lung cancer is supported by her daughter:

> *Interviewer:* Did you have anything else that could have ... flagged as a risk factor to the doctor? Did you smoke or anything that they would have picked up on?
>
> *Patient:* Smoked yeah. I did smoke.
>
> *Interviewer:* And did they ask you about that?
>
> *Patient:* Yeah, hmmm. It's something that I've done, it's very wrong.
>
> *Partner:* [Sternly] Do you know mum it's not the smoking that's the issue, we were discussing the GP here. ... we're not judging you at all. (52, lung cancer, interview 1, patient and partner)

This notion of personal responsibility is entwined with other dominant cultural messages about cancer that have been subsumed into understandings of aetiology. One element that several speakers noted was the ageing process and increased risk. Participants in the study drew on this in explaining their disease, demonstrating their received understanding of medical knowledge. Age is invoked by the next speaker, indicating its prevalence in mediating the experience of cancer. For this speaker, she felt as though others would not perceive her to have cancer because of her relative youthfulness:

> *Interviewer:* Why do you think they thought that, that you couldn't be a
> cancer patient?
> *Patient:* I think because I'm young, I think because when you go in there
> and I mean and most people are, are not, or even people like, who are
> maybe my age that don't, their mother will drive them in and things
> like that as well, you know so quite often, eh, there's like a girl she's, she
> was in the slot after me and her mum drove her in, so she was a young
> girl like me, but she was going with a sort of grey-haired old lady so
> they were ... probably just thought ... it's probably the grey-haired old
> lady, you know just [...] in some ways I kind of want to go round and
> say, say hello, and, and help to tell people ... because I just, like I want
> acknowledgement for it or something like that. (70, breast cancer, interview 2;
> patient only)

Culture was also invoked as people spoke about the meaning of Scottishness as part of their experience of cancer. This was an idea linked with a difficulty in expressing emotion, and was expressed alongside a clearly gendered experience. One man, the partner of someone with lung cancer, flippantly expresses how this is compared with his response to the death of the TV character from the *Waltons*: 'There's a whole lot more laughter than, than, than there is em, tears and, the tears come and the thing for me being a pretty you know, Scottish male, I think the last time I cried was probably when grandma Walton died' (69; lung cancer, interview 1, patient and partner). A further respondent talks about his view of pain control and how this is mediated by his culture and gendered ideas about expressing discomfort:

> Em, and but there was a few you know like, em, one, one girl there's a
> chemist so you know, she was saying to me, when I, my bones ached and my
> joints ached, she says take the 'ibuprofen and the paracetamol as well,' you
> know, so she, so but, you don't like to go on about it because you know, know
> what I mean, if your not, it must be a British thing or a Scottish thing – you
> just don't moan, when people say to 'are you alright,' you say 'OK, I'm fine,
> yeah I'm fine' and that was the way we were brought up, my mum used to
> say, 'don't tell, don't ...' [laughs]. (42, gynaecological cancer, interview 2, patient only)

Thus cultural scripts around ageing, gender, Scottishness, tobacco and changing norms about the appropriateness of discussing cancer are all demonstrated as pertinent to how people understand and relate to cancer. Alongside culture are religious and spiritual belief systems, which arbitrate people's understandings of cancer. As noted above, the dominance of one level over another can change and shift, thus, religious beliefs may subsume cultural contexts or vice versa.

Religion and spiritual beliefs

Several of the study's participants invoked notions of religiosity and spirituality to account for the occurrence of cancer or their adaptive coping style of acceptance of the course of ill health. Religion was often drawn upon in people's accounts, and was used by speakers to construct strength in the face of coping with the adversity of cancer: 'I go to a prayer meeting and they pray for me at that prayer meeting and eh, also within the, when our communions that we've brought up as well, and just the fact that you've got prayer and you've got all these people who believe ...' (42, gynaecological cancer, interview 2, patient only). Later this same speaker suggests that her faith provides a support and that other secular people may get this from counselling:

> The nurse said that she thought that we could do with counselling because I had lost my mum ... as well ... em, but nothing followed through from that and I didn't follow it through ... and I said to [husband], weeks later, I said 'I feel I'm coping with this.' Also, I've got faith as well, he's not a Christian and I am, so, I said to him, 'do you not, do you think you would need counselling?' (42, gynaecological cancer, interview 2, patient only)

Faith is invoked then as a way of explaining and providing strength. Another woman contextualises her experience and response in terms that construct her religious identity as a feature of coping: 'Well I'm not, I'm not religious in religious but it's just, I think because of things like that, I think I've probably prayed more in this last sort of few weeks than I have in my life!' (70, breast cancer, interview 1, patient only). Another woman, who described herself as a spiritualist, explains the belief system that creates the context for her experience of cancer and identifies her belief system as a place where she draws strength:

> *Patient:* My church does a lot of healing, you've probably heard of spiritualist healers, 'come to healing that will help' and emm they would put my name on the healing list because we pray for people to be healed every Sunday [...] I don't believe that I can expect [to] go through life unscathed, just because I can say I believe in God, you know, why should anything like that happen to me, these things happen. You're just part of the Earth.
> *Interviewer:* Mhmm, so when you think sort of ... 'Why me?' is your

answer, 'well these things happen,' 'cause you're part of Earth as you say ...?

Patient: I'm part of the Earth, and it may have come to teach me some lessons or give me some experience that I need.

Interviewer: Right and does that ... I was going to say, make you feel brave, but do you know, does it, does it help in terms of ...?

Patient: I feel very close to the spirit world, yes, so I feel that they're constantly around me and guiding me and supporting me. (10, breast cancer, interview 1, patient only)

The cause of cancer is therefore explained as something natural, part of the Earth, and which can not be protected against through faith or religiosity. Indeed, this belief system is used to account for the cancer as something she has experienced in order to 'teach' her some lessons. Such accounts contribute to a construction of cancer as something natural. For a very small number of participants, their religious belief systems were a higher organising context for understanding their cancer than medicine. This is a possible interpretation for Patient 10, above. This speaker explained further the role of her religious beliefs in her decision to not continue to take cancer medication:

I won't die before God wants me to die, so I don't think my life is in their [doctors] hands, I think it's in God's hands, you know. I'll live as long as He wants me to live, yeah. And isn't this an awful thing to say, I told this to my cousin and she was horrified, but I haven't got a great deal that I want to go on living for, I haven't got a husband, I haven't got children, I haven't got a family, I've finished with my career, I haven't got maybe the incentive that other people will take, to take horrible medicines in the hope that it'll keep them alive. (10, breast cancer, interview 2, patient only)

Thus, religion was a significant factor in the wider social context and experience of cancer for some individuals. It provided a mechanism for explaining ill health, and a network of supportive people and prayer. As the speaker above suggests, however, there may be competition between religion and the dominance of the medical model, where placing trust in God is more salient than physicians. However, for many participants the governing role of the medical team was unchallenged, and forms a significant feature of the experience of cancer.

Trust in professionals and the medical model

The views and attitudes of professionals played a significant role in how people subsequently related to their disease and the meanings they attached to it. Belief in individual professionals and the medical model was illustrated in many people's conversations, primarily as they accounted for how treatment decisions were made.

For the majority, there was a sense of relying on professionals to take the expert position and to guide the choice of suitable treatments and viewing medical personnel as imbued with higher levels of knowledge and expertise. However, a sizeable minority did position themselves as lay experts. The following couple jointly constructed the idea of deferring to medical expertise and fate epitomising how people spoke about treatment decision-making:

> *Patient:* I just left it to him [the consultant]. I didn't think.
> *Interviewer:* Why did you just leave it to him?
> *Patient:* I just think, I just thought … that he knew that, he knew what he was doing. Maybe I didn't know enough to ask a question either. You know.
> *Partner:* And you didn't, you went in with the thought of well 'what's going to be is, going to be'.
> *Patient:* Aha.
> *Partner:* And maybe too much knowledge is a bad thing for a lay person. If it's got to be dealt with, it's got to be dealt with. (61, breast cancer, interview 1, patient and partner)

The privileging of medical knowledge is dominant in this couple's view and was reinforced throughout interviews with professionals. Professionals at times identified patients as not being able to take an expert position on their illness, leaving treatment decision-making up to the clinicians:

> I would say, not being derogatory to lung cancer patients, the majority of patients will still take any decision that the medical staff offer them, they will be told that, you know, we've had a multidisciplinary meeting, the option that we think has a, as a professional team that the best is this, but that obviously they don't have to take that choice, but sadly in lung cancer, choices are limited. (63, lung cancer, clinical nurse specialist)

The sheer complexity of the physiology, anatomy and pathology meant that for many people, prioritising medical knowledge seemed like an unquestionable response. People referred to cancer centres as being 'world renowned' and therefore unquestionable in the expertise that professionals hold:

> I don't think there was any decision on my part that was their treatment. As far as I am concerned, if you have got a broken leg you stick a plaster on it, if you've got this then you get whatever they tell. And I am quite happy to go along with them as the experts and their knowledge and training, whatever. (01, colorectal cancer, interview 1, patient and partner)

For several people, the experience of cancer was in the context of having a professional clinical role themselves, or having close family members who were clinically trained. For the following speaker, this clearly impacts upon how they made sense of their diagnosis and expectations for treatment:

> *Interviewer:* Now that you've, you've had cancer you've had your treat-
> ments and surgery, has it made you think differently about what cancer
> is and, and what happens to people and their families, when somebody
> has cancer?
>
> *Patient:* I don't know if it's made much difference I, I was a nurse and I
> nursed a lot of people with cancer you know and I mean I know what
> they went through and I know what their families went through, so I've
> a good idea what it, what could happen. (54, breast cancer, interview 2, patient
> only)

The above speaker was asked specifically to reflect on how she relates to cancer, with a driving hypothesis that a personal experience of the disease will have shifted its meaning in someway. The patient replies that their professional role as a nurse had prepared them for 'what could happen'.

Changing relationships with the medical profession and with cancer have led to many people affected by cancer taking on a more assertive role in their care path-ways, not just for people who hold dual identities as nurses and people with cancer. One daughter clearly documented her role in managing her relationship with the medical professionals: 'I grilled them and you know I said to them you know, "Well she's [mother] skinny enough as it is, does she really have to go through the chemo, is there not any alternative treatments?" We went down every avenue you know and they were really good. They were straightforward and that's what mum wanted' (06, colorectal cancer interview 2, patient and partner). Another patient revealed how they were supported by clinicians to develop an informed stance with which to decide upon appropriate treatment choices: 'They told me to have a look at the book and read about the different choices and then when I had to go back they would talk about it in front of the consultant' (04, prostate cancer, interview 1, patient and partner).

Beliefs about the medical model and professional expertise were dominant ways in which people contextualised and explained their responses to cancer. The majority of people affected by cancer deferred to the clinicians' medical knowledge in deciding upon treatments. However, running alongside the medical model was a powerful way of explaining cancer's aetiology and prognosis linked with family experiences. Thus, again the contextual influences dance to privilege not God or the doctor in understanding how people relate to cancer, but their own family experiences.

Family scripts and family beliefs

With cancer affecting one in three people over the life course, it is rare to find someone who does not have a familial experience of cancer. For participants in this study, drawing on family scripts and experiences of cancer formed an important mechanism for organising and explaining their own experience. The notion of 'family scripts' is reminiscent of metaphors of theatre. Scripts have been defined as part of a sequence of interactions and transactions around specific events, whereby individuals learn how to react and respond (Byng-Hall, 1985). They provide 'ready guidance for action' (Byng-Hall, 1985: 303), and connect generations, since each individual takes their parents' script and blends it into a new one. Over time families may try and 'correct' a script that has gone awry in previous generations. In the context of cancer, this may be a family script about its terminality or symptom morbidity.

For some people affected by cancer, the dominance of family scripts or family beliefs were paramount in mediating their experience and understanding of the disease. For these individuals, the family script was the dominant context through which their cancer was experienced and understood. There was a sense that family experiences of cancer outweighed the medical views of prognosis:

> My son and daughter they don't see anything realistic signs of any demise on my behalf. They just think 'well you've been told he could last for five years' and I said, I didn't tell them that at all, I says that 'if I don't get treatment, people who don't get treatment seventy-two per cent of them will live five years and those who do seventy-two per cent will live five years'. They thought 'oh well this is great. You've been told you don't need it so you can still live five years.' It doesn't work out that way. As I say it depends how virulent these damn things are. How quick it can take you out. They won't accept that. She's just lost her uncle to cancer and she won't accept that he's dead. (33, colorectal cancer, interview 1, patient only)

The interplay of different social contexts can be seen as being played out here as medical and statistical ideas of demise are set against family scripts. The loss of an uncle to cancer seems to have played a role in inoculating the children from internalising a worrying prognosis. This is further reinforced with more explicit contrasts between medical and family understandings of health, and connects with the discussion in Chapter 8 around comorbid conditions:

> I'm not concerned. As I say, the poor doctor sitting there, he was more worried than I am. And I said to him, you know he said 'does it concern you what I've told you?' I said 'no'. I said 'men in my family don't die of cancer, they drop down dead of heart attacks.' But it's going to be a race to which one takes me out first. (33, colorectal cancer, interview 1, patient only)

For some individuals, the diagnosis of cancer was experienced as expected, with participants indicating that they had many relatives who had also had the disease. Cancer was a dominant part of these people's family life-cycles and so was considered an intergenerational illness. Many participants mentioned cancer as a predictable and expected part of family life and age-related health transitions. However, having an expectation and awareness of susceptibility did not always protect against the shock of being given a diagnosis:

> I had no idea that it would be malignant … but there was always a chance of that. I mean that was still at the back of my mind, I suppose, really, because my father … he didn't die of that, but it was present … he was 83 when he died. It was discovered when he was in hospital, and again he may have had it for some considerable time … we didn't really think there would be any real problem … (19, prostate cancer, interview 1, patient only)

The association between cancer and death was often also cited in the context of a family script. Despite the innocuous question about reading up on cancer, the following description of family experiences of cancer is the speaker's very powerful response:

> *Interviewer:* What is it you've been reading about cancer?
> *Patient:* I've read a lot about cancer up and down because my eldest brother died of cancer. He went off to his bed on the Saturday night because his family had a meal that night because they were all in a crowd, but he wasn't able to go and when they come home his daughter says 'oh my God.' Dad had says 'I'll need to go back and see what's to do'. He was dead, but something burst and he bled to death. The bed and the carpet they had to throw anything out. Full of blood. So I wouldn't like that to happen to me. I don't know, no idea, but that was his and it was cancer that he had. (20, gynaecological cancer, interview 2, patient only)

Healthcare professionals reinforced the notion of family scripts as an important factor in people's experience of expecting, but still being shocked by, the diagnosis: 'She was actually very shocked at the time when she was told. I think having had a family history of breast cancer she knows there is always a chance there that we will find something. And what was told to her at the time was that we had found this small cancer in her breast, that it was treatable' (05, breast cancer, clinical nurse specialist).

A man with prostate cancer told of his extensive family history of cancer, including his grandfather, father, brother and other relatives. For him, and many others, cancer was a predicted component to life, and considered a normal part of the family's health trajectory. Indeed, he employed a strategy pre-diagnosis to cope with the possibility of developing prostate cancer by having six monthly prostate specific antigen tests. 'Why me? Because it's in my genes. As far as I'm concerned I know it's in the genes somewhere. It's just a matter of where it might appear or what form it's going to take and do something about it as soon as it's observed' (62, prostate cancer, interview 1 patient only). The speaker imputes the inevitable appearance of cancer to a genetic susceptibility. However, although this may reduce the threat of its existence in his life, it does not lessen the implications and impact in terms of treatment. He perceives the latter as major disruption, a perception informed by previously caring for a friend with prostate cancer:

> And the only thing one worries about is not the cancer but the treatment …
> I was taking him to the hospital and I was sharing all this experience with
> him which he ultimately, although he had wonderful care but ultimately
> it's a very stressful, unpleasant experience … he had this horrific, eh, this
> treatment … chemotherapy. And I mean it really knocked him out. Very
> unpleasant. (62, prostate cancer, interview one, patient only)

This experience, combined with his knowledge of the possible implications of chemotherapy, had a clear impact on his well-being. Such experiences informed his
decision-making around treatment, leading him to choose brachytherapy over other
treatments.

Family scripts were closely linked with biological and genetic understandings.
Again these form contexts in which cancer is experienced in the present, as well as
extending out to the past and forward into the future. One woman with a gynaecological cancer speaks about her family's experiences of cancer:

> People have told me that it's mainly your genes, I've been told that it's in
> your genes and that worries with my granddaughters you know what I
> mean? That's the only thing I can think of. When they told me that it's
> an ovarian cancer and usually it's carried in genes so it's like inherited off
> your family, I can remember my nan dying and her belly was like a lady
> that was pregnant but at the time I didn't realise, so it looks like they are
> right in that way it is something that's in your genes and that you've got to
> be aware of and perhaps in the future that they will be able to turn round
> and people that it is in the genes that they can spot it quicker and they can
> do something to help them. As I said I've got granddaughters and I think
> to myself I'd hate them to have to come to this if it can be spotted sooner
> and put right and they can have a better life. (65, gynaecological cancer, interview
> 2, patient only)

Healthcare professionals recognised the importance of family scripts about cancer
and family support: 'It's quite interesting 'cause em, her father died of cancer of the
oesophagus when she was a very young child, so mother brought up four kids on her
own and they're, they're a very fine family, they're mutually supportive, you know,
and always have been and they were all very much through this, and she stays with
her mum' (09, gynaecological cancer, GP). Thus, cancer has occurred within the context of a
wealth of family experiences of cancer and other conditions. These understandings
form part of the ways in which cancer is understood – it is not a unique one-off occurrence, but has come into people's lives with a legacy. Throughout the interviews,
cancer was presented as connected to other people's lives, and to others' symptoms,
coping, recovery and decline.

Episodes

Sitting within and alongside each of the contextual layers indicated above are individual episodes – instances where cancer is brought to the fore for an individual by a particular incident. The meanings given to these episodes are influenced by the higher levels of context and illustrate the movement of different explanations and frameworks. The following interview extracts illustrate the interplay of contextual layers and how meaning shifts and moves for speakers, as they construct their account of cancer and its impact on their life. The speakers link individual scripts with medical and spiritual dimensions, illustrating this dynamic interplay of contextual layers:

> *Patient:* It would be nice if there was someone who specifically talked to patients about what to expect.
>
> *Partner:* I suppose [the Macmillan nurse] does that to an extent.
>
> *Patient:* [She] does that but you would like to know it whilst you're in hospital and undergoing, well to begin with you can't, I mean if you've just been operated on then I should imagine they're not awfully sure whether you're going to make it or not in a lot of cases. But during that period of time there should be someone there who can come and talk to patients. It's all very well the chaplain coming and chatting to you, the minute you see her you think oh my God. Hail Mary full of grace. Em …
>
> *Partner:* You think they've got a measuring tape in their pocket, you know.
>
> (40, gynaecological cancer, interview 2, patient and partner)

A similar effect of leaping between important contextual layers that guide meaning-making is created by the following speaker's description of her own cancer. She joins the medical model (including her own professional role) with a family script about what it means to personally experience cancer:

> *Patient:* Well, I have to say the hardest bit of the whole thing for me has been, I think, as a nurse, I've always been quite, well maybe not as a nurse, just in general, I think I've always been quite judgemental in my own mind about people who get cancer, and I have to say my brother died three years ago from pancreatic cancer, so it would apply all my thoughts about him as well, you now, and what I perceive cancer people to be like. I suppose I think of them as people who, em, harbour all their feelings and maybe don't, you know... [my brother] was quite sacrificing wasn't he in his own way, he put everybody first and, em you know his ex-wife died of a brain tumour and they had a son so [my brother] had the son full time and you know didn't always do all the things he wanted to do I don't think and …
>
> *Mother:* And his partner who …
>
> *Patient:* Yes, who caused a lot of sort of problems because of her, she

> couldn't deal with the son and all those things. So I think I was even applying these, you know, and then you get these lovely old ladies who'd come in who wouldn't say boo to anybody and 'no I'm fine just you leave me, sort me out when you get time'. Sort of martyr-ish I suppose, and a bit, I don't like to say it, but kind of door mat-ish like and I always think well, I vent my spleen don't I? (55, breast cancer, interview 1, patient and mother)

Notions of blame are wrapped up with the medical model, as people who develop cancer are, at times, constructed as responsible for their own disease. This patient reflects on her own belief system about her brother's martyred life, but juxtaposes this against her own approach of expressing her emotions (venting her spleen). The shift of organising contexts is deftly accomplished so she is not asked to account for her own self-responsibility for ill health.

For the following speaker, her own episode of cancer is explored alongside culturally available ideas of the genetic transmission of cancer, alongside smoking as a carcinogen. This, as with the previous extract, evokes ideas of responsibility and self-blame for ill health.

> *Patient:* I should probably add that my mother died about five, six years ago at (age) eight-four, eighty-five. She died with lung cancer but that was put down to smoking. But she was kind of well past her sell-by date by that time. Although she again was another clean-living woman, never went out you know, things like that but, a smoking problem with her. I'm just hoping there's not a gene there you know. Maybe not.
> *Interviewer:* Are you exploring that possibility?
> *Patient:* No I'm not. I told you I'm blanking it out. For whatever reason that I, I'm just not facing the reality sorry but it's the way I'm feeling you know. My reaction when it happened, oh that's not me, I'll waken up tomorrow it'll go away you know. I didn't expect this' (46, lung cancer, interview 1, patient and partner)

For this speaker and the ones who go before, there is a delicate interplay of different contextual layers, from broad social discourses of cancer, through to individualised ones around family scripts. Each of these provide ways of accounting for and making sense of an individual and unique episode of cancer in their lives.

Summary

Coordinated Management of Meaning has been applied as a framework to unpick the different and competing contexts in which cancer is understood, and how people organise their accounts of ill health with regard to different contextual forces.

By looking at the different contextual layers in which cancer is experienced, it becomes possible to understand some of the complexities of living with the disease.

Cultural discourses impact upon the ways in which cancer is experienced, as something which is blameworthy and where there have been substantial shifts over time in how publicly people can speak of cancer. Intergenerational understandings of cancer and the socio-cultural climate are each played out in family scripts and individual episodes of cancer. Each of these has a recursive impact on cancer's influence and consequent levels of distress within family systems.

Considering the hierarchical contexts in which people experience cancer forces attention beyond the tumour and viewing cancer as an individual disease. This chapter has highlighted powerfully the interconnectedness between all parts of the system, and the consequent impact on the experience of cancer. The notion of layers is not intended to imply the peeling away of layers of an onion which leads to a hidden inner truth. Rather, the layers shift from moment to moment and are considered to hold competing explanatory powers that shed light on how people experience and relate to their cancers.

Chapter 10

Implications and applications

This book has unashamedly presented evidence that supports a move toward a more complex and nuanced understanding of what it means to experience cancer. Its essence is the need to understand cancer in the context of its fullest impact on the people affected by the disease. This chapter outlines a systemic approach to ill health and expedites policy implications and practice applications of adopting a systemic approach to cancer care. This approach goes beyond the traditional policy and practice models, including patient-centred care, patient experiences, partnership working and carers' roles and rights. It is a call for practitioners, in particular, to think and act in a way that is mindful of systemic theory and practice and the intricacies of interrelationships and social context.

The book has explored different layers and components of the social contexts of cancer, illustrating how cancer does not exist in a void. Cancer itself also forms a context for experience, that is, it reframes and situates experiences of relationships, professional interactions, employment and identity. Better cancer care must take account of the various contexts in which the disease is experienced, and how the disease affects these contexts. Chapters about families and professionals lay the groundwork for this approach, by identifying the ways in which people affected by cancer reflect upon these key relationships as central components to, and mediators of, their experience of cancer. Relationships with other patients were explored to highlight the role that others with direct experiential knowledge of the illness have on people's views of their own direct and personal experience of cancer. The complexities of cancer in the face of employment have been explored to begin to broaden out reflections on the systems that are affected by cancer. The physical sequelae of cancer has been noted in several chapters taking, at times, a sideways look at the traditional territory of cancer as a physical disease and positioning cancer as something that people externalise and relate to. The book also examined the wider identity work that people affected by cancer engage in, to manage how they view themselves and how others view them in relation to cancer. The previous chapter explored the contextual influences on constructed meanings of cancer, relating the biological, the social and cultural elements to the personal experience of the disease.

In this concluding chapter we highlight some of the conceptual issues that are pivotal to a systemic framework. We draw exclusively on our study of people's experience of cancer although we believe that it is a framework that can be used for understanding experiences of a range of conditions.

A systemic framework

This book has focused on the experiences of people with cancer and of those who they interact with, including family members, health professionals, friends and neighbours. It draws attention to cancer as an illness that is mediated by different contexts and is defined and made sense of through processes of negotiation with others. The systemic approach looks not only at the individual with the disease but the wider socio-cultural spaces in which cancer is experienced and related to.

Cancer can be investigated and treated as a biological phenomenon; it has a molecular existence and can be studied and treated as such. In contrast to medical models of illness that have focused on the disease, the systemic approach focuses on the people affected by the disease, the context in which the disease is experienced and the meanings associated with the illness. Challenges to, and augmentations of, medical-model thinking have been developed within the social sciences. Social science approaches have a lengthy legacy, for example, of situating health and illness within socio-historical contexts (Foucault, 1977; Foucault, 2006). The move toward person-centred care has also provided a challenge to the medical model, and operates with an assumption that *individuals* are the unit of (medical) concern and (research) analysis. Although more satisfying than a purely medical model, person-centred models still struggle to make sense of the wider relational contexts in which illness is experienced.

The approach described and illustrated in this book however is substantially different to, and is a more sophisticated model than one which is traditionally drawn upon to understand the impacts of illness. Systemic approaches to illness stress that the patient is not just playing host to a tumour, but experiences cancer in the wider context of their lives. It is this relational and context-aware approach that health professionals must be mindful of as part of their duty of care.

Systemic approaches, applied most frequently in family therapy practice contexts, can be traced back to a number of theorists who have drawn together a range of academic disciplines to understand human behaviour and experience. Bateson (1973), for example, is identified as one of the founding thinkers in systemic theory; drawing his ideas from a disparate range of disciplines such as anthropology, biology and psychiatry. At its heart, Bateson's approach argues that a systemic framework must be mindful of the total ecology in mediating experience. One core tenet is that a change in one part of the system (such as the diagnosis of an illness) leads to changes in other parts of the system (for example, relatives may feel pulled into the family system in the centripetal style described in Chapter 3). The approach then argues that experience is a complex phenomenon, and that the context in which cancer occurs will mediate the meanings and significances attached to it. This disrupts a linear construction of the impact of cancer on people, and takes into account the recursive and iterative forces between cancer, relationships and social context.

The term *system* can be taken to mean a range of different layers and levels for example: family, work, society. In contemporary practice, the idea that change in one part of a system leads to other changes is exemplified in the belief that individuals and their behaviours cannot be dissociated from their relational and social contexts. Thus, to understand cancer, or other illnesses, there is a need to move beyond disease models and looking at individuals, to seeing people as interconnected with others and the wider socio-cultural environment. A systemic approach therefore asserts that the whole is more than the sum of its parts and can only be truly understood when it is viewed in its complex state.

Thus, this book serves to extend the analytic lens beyond the individual level by focusing on the relationship and social context as mediating meaning and experience. This is relatively new terrain within cancer care research, and builds on the work of others looking at healthcare with a systemic lens, such as (Rolland, 1994; Rolland, 1999), by providing research-based evidence about the utility of the approach.

The purpose of this chapter is to articulate our understanding of the systemic approach by drawing on, and in response to, the wealth of data that are presented in preceding chapters. The data provide an opportunity to highlight key themes characteristic of a systemic approach that are visible in the experiences of people affected by cancer.

We intend a systemic approach as both a descriptive and explanatory device. That is, we wish to describe ill health within contexts and particular relationships, *and* we wish to use social interactions and connectivity with others to explain experiences of ill health.

The following sections synthesise some of the key issues around rethinking the delivery of cancer care that come about through adopting a systemic approach.

Theme one: The impact of cancer on relationships

As we have argued in the preceding chapters, cancer impacts upon a range of systems and relationships. Although a physical illness such as cancer is located within one person, its impact reaches far beyond that individual. As with a range of acute and chronic conditions, a diagnosis of cancer affects not just the individual who has the disease but is experienced by a wide network of people. Relatives, friends and colleagues will all be affected. Family members and close friends may experience emotional strain, financial loss arising from caring and changes in their relationships. Thus, people who have proximity to the patient may also have health and social needs as a consequence of the impact of ill health. Indeed, there is a growing body of evidence concerning the psychological health and well-being of unpaid carers/significant others of people with cancer (Kim *et al.*, 2006). However, such approaches stop short of what we are proposing with systemic theories. We suggest a need to look at cancer relationally, not solely separating patient from carer, but viewing the relationship itself as being impacted on and as part of the mediating process of understanding the experience of the disease. Further, we contend that the relationship itself can be the unit care. That is, the patient–family member relationship could readily be the focus of statutory services' support.

The role that others play in practical and emotional terms has been described at length in the preceding chapters, and it is most evident within families. Current policy recognises the central role of relatives and other informal carers in supporting people with cancer (NICE, 2004; Scottish Executive, 2005a; Scottish Executive, 2005b; Scottish Executive, 2007). Our study clearly marks out changing roles for partners of people with cancer, plainly indicating the impact of cancer beyond the diagnosed patient.

In the past, accounts of the role of others would be described in terms of unidirectional caregiving, with implications of dependency. The book recognises the value of the interdependencies and reciprocity in relationships where someone is unwell (Brechin *et al.*, 1998). The notion of reciprocity that is now integrated into academic theorising around care, however, stops short of the systemic approach to practice. It separates out carer from patient, rather than seeking to identify the role of the relationship and context as the site of cancer experience. Reciprocity theories are systemic only in as much as reciprocity recognises the interconnections between different people; however it does not reflect a core idea that change in one part of the system leads to changes in other parts. The evidence for a systemic approach to understanding the role of others is demonstrated, for example, in Chapter 3, as people with cancer chose to protect relatives from their diagnosis and the full implications and ramifications of the disease. Ill health can be seen to threaten disruption to people's positions within the family. Partners faced with illness may, for example, renegotiate their role as the main financial provider or as the main provider of housework. The data clearly demonstrate that it was not unusual for either the person with cancer or their friends/relatives to provide support to each other in financial, practical and emotional terms, requiring a renegotiation of a range of tasks and roles. A well rehearsed debate of the shift in role from 'wife/husband' to carer is evoked here, as people position themselves within the shifting relational sands that ill health has brought.

Notable in its absence from the data was a sense that partners of those with the illness felt included in the provision of services and development of a meaningful relationship with healthcare professionals. This seems at odds with the abundance of policy relating to informal carers (OPM *et al.*, 2006) and the drivers to provide services to support in their role providing unpaid care. This is particularly noteworthy given the strong sense of joint ownership of the disease by the person with the cancer *and* their partner. Constructing cancer to be a shared experience was keenly visible in the data, yet this understanding does not appear to inform professionals' approaches to care.

The implications for improved cancer care are in taking on a more nuanced approach to understanding the role of others in mediating the experience of cancer and how cancer impacts upon relationships. The actions of relatives, friends and colleagues are all critical to developing a systemic approach where the interconnections are better understood and cancer can be seen to impact on relationships. Healthcare professionals who are mindful of the impact of cancer upon relationships will be able to make a small but significant conceptual shift toward a systemic approach to cancer care.

Theme two: The impact of relationships on the experience of cancer

The family can be considered both a resource and a recipient of the impact of a serious diagnosis. The previous section reflected on the impact of cancer on relationships; this section inverts the supposition, positioning relationships as having an impact upon cancer. A systemic approach highlights that family dynamics and relationships play a part in both how the disease is related to and the overall (ill) health experience.

Relationships between professionals and people affected by cancer impact on the experience of cancer. Relationships have long been considered to be the process of care and the vehicle for recovery in psychological disciplines (Lambert and Barley, 2001), an assertion which can be seen as fitting neatly with experiences of a cancer diagnosis. Exploring relationships between professionals and patients in cancer care has traditionally focused on communication and information provision (Shilling *et al.*, 2003). This book has drawn attention to the significance of how cancer affects relationships with health professionals in a slightly different way by looking at how relationships themselves impact upon the experience of cancer, and access to services.

Even with recent shifts toward recognising patient expertise in their own experience (Department of Health, 2001), the views and actions of professionals still loom large in the overall experience of cancer and people's relationships to it. For example, a practitioner's views on the disease often shapes the patient's and partner's views about the aggressiveness of the cancer; likewise professionals who make themselves available to patients foster a situation in which worries can be raised and discussed. Further, the data highlight how important relationships between professionals and people affected by cancer are in determining service use. The reticence of people requesting services from GPs or community nurses, for example, illustrates the impact of the relationship in leading to differential access to services. In each instance cited above, the relationship between professionals and people affected by cancer impact on how the disease is experienced.

Both patients and partners reported their views on how they wished professionals to adopt particular behaviours and relationships with them. Courtesy calls from GPs, regular contact with community nurses and other signifiers of a tailored approach to care were named. This gave them a sense that they were treated as a person living in a range of contexts and systems, not just the unfortunate host of a biological disease.

Subtle non-verbal communications from professionals also impact on how people experienced cancer. Non-verbal cues were understood, at times, as signifying a worrying diagnosis or prognosis. The cultural backdrop of viewing cancer as a worrying, and often fatal, disease therefore also contributed to the complex interplay of how people affected by cancer related to healthcare professionals. Overall, the data underline the critical role that healthcare professionals play in how cancer was experienced and related to. Healthcare professionals would do well to scrutinise their own belief systems around ill health, including reflection on their own familial experiences and understanding of the wider socio-political contexts. The effect of such an exercise would be to identify how views mediate their ideas about cancer and approaches to people affected by cancer.

Notable at times was the limited interaction between professionals and partners or other family members despite their need of support. Such compartmentalisation is perhaps understandable in terms of professionals' workloads, but exposes care delivery as giving inadequate recognition to the relationships between individuals and the importance of these to recovery.

The family and other relationships are also a vehicle for managing and experiencing cancer. Using family or informal support networks is often constructed in policy terms as informal/unpaid care. Indeed, family members have been widely heralded as the lynchpin of modern care systems. This has been taken up by healthcare professionals to some extent. For example, professionals at times encourage patients to invite a family member or friend to appointments, to provide emotional support and practical help in processing information (Hubbard *et al.*, 2009b). Such changes in practice indicate the growing uptake of the idea that relationships are important.

One of the clear ways in which relationships impact upon the meaning and experience of cancer is through successive generations within families. Multigenerational patterns of cancer experiences go beyond the genetic heritability of disease and butt up against family folklore and accounts of illness, treatment and prognosis. Life-cycle stages of individuals and of the family (such as teenage years and retirement) also play a role in altering how cancer is related to and the recursive impact with family systems. Similarly, the experiences of friends, colleagues and communities will feed into people's understandings of cancer as a death sentence or an opportunity for reassessing core beliefs and values and augmenting changes to identity. Other people with experiences of cancer play important roles in providing experientially based expert knowledge about the disease and its consequences. Yet in reality such experience is given little credence within the development of cancer services. Although recent policy (Scottish Government, 2008; Scottish Government, 2009) extols the value of patient experience, translating this into meaningful engagement of people affected by cancer remains an elusive goal.

Family members identified themselves as having a key role in encouraging the person with cancer to seek initial appointments and tests leading to diagnosis. Relatives took on a range of practical, physical and emotional tasks, often beginning before the diagnosis. For instance, the identity work within partner narratives across the interviews constructs a polarity, where family members take up a position around timely diagnosis, whereas primary care physicians are implicated more often in delayed diagnosis. The triadic relationship between patient, partner and primary care team therefore plays a central role in the family accounts around diagnosis and how symptoms were communicated and managed.

Building relationships between each part of the triad (healthcare professional, patient and partner) was considered to be a critical component of better cancer care. This shifts the focus away from conventional approaches that treat each in isolation, and adopts a systemic approach which focuses at a relational level.

Family and wider relationships, and accounts of illness, therefore impact upon how cancer itself is understood. Professionals are likely to miss this nuanced contextualisation of the phenotypic expression and experience of cancer if they attend only to the disease process.

The importance of supporting families has been clearly acknowledged in Government programmes such as the *Think Family* approach to social care (Cabinet Office and Social Exclusion Task Force, 2007). This document encourages services to prioritise family well-being, and provide support to families identifying the multigenerational impact of complex lives: 'When parents experience difficulties in their own lives, the impact can be severe and enduring for both themselves and for their children. The consequences can cast a shadow that spans whole lifetimes' (Cabinet Office and Social Exclusion Task Force, 2007: 7).

Although the *Think Family* initiative is structured around families with young children, the core tenet of it has salience to those without. The identified approach could equally be applied to adult cancer care: 'Tailored, flexible and holistic services that work with the whole family can turn lives around dramatically' ((Cabinet Office and Social Exclusion Task Force, 2007: 4).

Better cancer care must be cognisant of the important role that relationships have in mediating the experience of the disease. Health and social policy must begin to build upon the work conducted in children's services, and embed relationship-based ideals in policy initiatives (Henderson and Forbat, 2002). This would mean moving beyond simplistic constructions of 'carer', to a position where cancer is understood as a disease whose impact is felt throughout entire relationship networks. Policy and practice should recognise, and provide support to, the multiple people who are affected by cancer. This would mean offering constructions of identities not just as patients or carers, but as people who jointly 'own' the experience, who legitimately claim it to have an important impact on them.

The idea of relationship-based social policy has been discussed across a range of conditions and needs for health care (Forbat, 2008; Henderson and Forbat, 2002), and is not limited to cancer. People's understandings of cause, heritability, fear of recurrence and prognosis all intersect to produce a climate that may have similarities to other chronic diseases such as dementia, heart disease, diabetes and motor neurone disease. Thus, a systemic approach, which is mindful of relationships within and beyond the family may be applicable to other diseases which occupy similar socio-cultural spaces.

Theme three: relating to cancer

Cancer has developed its own identity within society, which has shifted and morphed over the last twenty years. Treatment advances, in hand with media coverage, show that surviving cancer is more commonplace than it once was. As a consequence people's relationship to cancer has changed, from one of almost certain fatality to an understanding that it could be an acute condition requiring treatment, or a chronic disease which will continue to have repercussions for years to come. The social construction of cancer, thereby plays an important role in how people relate to it, and its subsequent impact on their experience of cancer.

Recent health policy has reinforced a number of messages about how people relate to cancer and its causes. In particular, bans on smoking in enclosed public spaces play a role in positioning cancer as something that people have a personal responsibility and personal liability for. Previous chapters have highlighted how people affected by cancer have actively created boundaries between themselves and the disease, by constructing cancer as an external entity to themselves. In some ways this is isomorphic to the medical model, separating tumour from individual. When people affected by cancer externalise the disease, however, the consequence is to construct cancer as self-determining and outside of the self. This externalising of cancer addresses the social context of blame and responsibility discourses, and enables people to reassert their relationship with the disease.

Study participants often related to, and experienced, cancer in the context of other comorbid conditions, which shaped their reactions to the cancer diagnosis and subsequent treatment and prognosis. Notions of biographical disruption or second-order changes to identity were called forth as people make sense of cancer in the context of other health conditions. Much as cancer is a context of experience, other illnesses also form contexts for understanding the experience of cancer care.

Indeed, the experience of other conditions may coalesce for the person and enable them to form a template and map with which to navigate the effects of cancer on self and others.

Professionals relate to cancer in a somewhat different manner to the participants who had a personal experience of cancer. Professionals relate to the disease as something that may require treatment and which ceases to have salient implications beyond active treatment. For people affected by cancer, the disease was often perceived as having much more salience in their lives, extending beyond treatment and often predicted to go beyond the five years following diagnosis, particularly for people taking tamoxifen. As noted above, opportunities for professionals to reflect on their own relationship with cancer, as informed by their own familial experiences and perceptions of the socio-cultural location of ill health will augment their ability to work systemically.

How people relate to the disease necessarily impacts upon its significance in their lives, and is therefore an important part of a systemic approach. Practitioners aiming to enhance cancer care should be mindful of the complex interplay of how people relate to their disease and how this will be different to professionals' views, as a consequence of their experiential knowledge and family circumstances. People can and do relate to cancer in a range of ways, which create the contexts for how it is experienced and what kind of care is required from professionals. Adopting a systemic approach to cancer care will mean that medical management of symptoms and side-effects shifts from a disease-based focus to one which is based upon a broader understanding of the context in which cancer is experienced.

Theme four: roles and relationships in society

One of the clear ways in which cancer has a social presence is through people's negotiation of employment during and following cancer. Employment was considered as one of the varied contexts which that organise identity, which subsequently impact on the meaning and consequence of disease. People who have been in employment throughout their lives may, when confronted with a cancer diagnosis, be unable to continue in their work. Consequently they may be compelled to renegotiate their identity as an employed member of society. This was evidenced when people who were close to retirement when diagnosed with cancer, decide to leave work early or when people were too ill to return to work.

The data highlight tensions between cancer and a range of other social responsibilities such pre-existing care roles. Healthcare professionals at times assisted people affected by cancer with welfare benefits claims, but this was a rare example of recognising people in their roles beyond being a cancer patient. This indicates the need for systemic understanding of people affected by cancer, as practitioners integrate disease knowledge into a more intricate appreciation of the complexities of people's lives and roles.

For example, to support people in managing the physical elements of cancer in their everyday lives, there is a need for practitioners to understand the context in which the illness is experienced. Treatment side-effects and ongoing medication are at present managed by the person with cancer and their family. Cancer care staff who have a role in supporting self-management and are interested in a systemic approach to practice should move towards an understanding of how this happens in the context of work and personal lives. For instance, managing nausea may be viewed in contemporary practice as a morbidity-related activity; systemic practice would involve a collaborative approach to managing the symptoms most bothersome to the people affected by cancer and coalesce around the most important issues for them. Nausea therefore is approached with the aim of facilitating the person's engagement in their preferred activities; it is no longer viewed narrowly as a physical side-effect of chemotherapy.

The concepts of partnership working and joined-up working are ubiquitous in Scotland's health policy documentation, and this is largely being implemented through the Managed Clinical Networks and Regional Cancer Advisory Groups. As the current policy direction of travel towards partnership gathers pace, other services and sectors have been brought into the healthcare planning and service delivery arena, including social care. Drawing on the data from this study, we argue that employment should be part of the partnership, because a large proportion of people affected by cancer require support and advice since their employment was affected as a consequence of having cancer.

Healthcare practitioners who recognise the importance of occupation for people with cancer are probably more likely to take steps to support those who wish to remain in work. For example, during treatment they may be able to discuss with an individual how to manage symptoms while being in work. Employers can also be supportive by taking steps to facilitate an individual who wishes to remain in work. This may involve formal and informal processes. An example of the latter is enabling the individual who is ill to pop in and out of the workplace although they are 'formally' either on sick leave or back at work full time.

Theme five: The presence of cancer across time and location

Two features concerning the presence of cancer across time warrant discussion. One is the longitudinal framing of the research data, which provides scope for exploring change over time. This is discussed in the context of short-term professional relationships with people affected by cancer. The second dimension relates to the intergenerational and societal transmission of beliefs across time, leading to changing relationships with cancer over time.

The study described in this book adopted a prospective, rather than cross-sectional, design. This enabled the plotting out of change and difference over time for each of the people involved. Longitudinal methods have been considered to be an appropriate method for systemic enquiry into ill health (Rolland, 1994) because they create possibilities for exploring the complexity of the impact of illness over time. This is a markedly different approach to understanding care than professionals tend to adopt. Services are organised and delivered in a fragmentary way, with divisions between primary, secondary and tertiary care facilities meaning that people affected by cancer see professionals as unlikely to have lengthy or sustained contact prior to diagnosis, through treatment and into follow-up care. This longitudinal approach also incorporates an understanding of change over generations. Adopting a systemic approach to cancer affords the opportunity to consider a range of dimensions such as the impact of family scripts and culturally available tropes that capture the sense and meaning of cancer. In this way, time is invoked as a pertinent dimension, as meanings shift and family stories around cancer evolve and shape people's relationship to the disease. Placing cancer in a temporal context also enables consideration of family and individual life-cycle stages, and the iterative relationship between experience of cancer and life stage. The appearance of cancer in a family at a time when teenagers are seeking further independence is experienced in a different way to cancer experienced in a family with adult (or no) children. Centrifugal and centripetal forces that draw people together or compel them to move apart will be influenced by life-stage developmental tasks. Further, an understanding of the impact of cancer over the course of time will enable the exploration of changing identities.

Although diagnosis is understood as a medical one-off event, the impact of the diagnosis and subsequent need for treatment and the experience of symptoms and side-effects may all have an ongoing effect. To understand more fully the experience of cancer, a systemic approach necessarily seeks to appreciate the identity journey that people engage in. This should move from prior to the identification of cancer (for example, a sense of self as healthy) through to treatment and then toward a self that is projected into the future (taking into account new future identity possibilities such as being infertile or with a much constricted life expectancy). As the previous chapters have illustrated, this impact on identity and sense of self is not limited to those individuals with the diagnosis of cancer, but has repercussions throughout a wide range of systems and relationships.

Cancer also has a presence across locations. Geography and diasporic relational networks mean that the influence of cancer extends beyond the immediate vicinity of close friends and relatives, to those living in different cities, countries and continents. Proximity to treatment centres and primary care facilities played a role too in how people experience their disease, and whether they felt more or less able to use statutory health care. Geographic landscapes therefore provide a relational architecture for shaping and influencing disease experiences between families, friends and healthcare professionals.

We argue that a longitudinal and temporal understanding of cancer for individuals and families is often missing from their professional understanding of the experience of cancer. People working in cancer care should integrate these dimensions of time and place into their practice. This means recognising the shifting meanings of cancer, of the temporality of their relationship with people affected by cancer and the impacts that geography has on accessing formal and informal support.

Developing a systemic approach to cancer care

The fact that cancer is a physical disease that requires specialist medical intervention is not disputed; but the dominance of the disease model is. Cancer is more than a disease entity, it can be life changing even if it is not considered life threatening in terms of disease pathology. Developing better cancer care should take stock of the myriad ways in which people affected by the disease experience it in the widest contexts of their lives.

This book, and the systemic approach described, is intended as an invitation to healthcare practitioners and policy makers to consider a shift in how they conceptualise care. At its heart, a systemic approach to enhancing cancer care is based on an understanding of the relational and contextual influences that impact upon the meaning of the disease, and the recursive loop connecting disease, relationships and contexts. The systemic approach requires shifting the gaze from the individual and the tumour to the social and relational contexts in which cancer occurs. In adopting this more nuanced appreciation of the disease's meaning comes a more refined understanding of the implications and ramifications of living with cancer for individuals, for families and across society.

References

Barber, J. (2002) 'The use of self', *Context*, June, pp. 2–7

Barge, J. K. (2004) 'Articulating CMM as a practical theory', *Human Systems*, Vol. 15, No. 3, pp. 193–204

Bateson, G. (1973) *Steps to an Ecology of Mind London*, New York: Paladin/Granada Publishing

Borkman, T. (1976) 'Experiential knowledge: A new concept for the analysis of self-help groups', *Social Services Review*, Vol. 50, No. 3, pp. 445–56

Boston, P. (2000) 'Systemic family therapy and the influence of post-modernism', *Advances in Psychiatric Treatment*, Vol. 6, No. 6, pp. 450–7

Brechin, A., Walmsley, J., Katz, J. and Peace, S. (1998) *Care Matters: Concepts, Practice and Research in Health and Social Care*, London: Sage

Burnham, J. (1986) *Family Therapy*, London: Sage

Burns, D. (2007) *Systemic Action Research: A strategy for whole system change*, Bristol: Policy Press

Bury, M. (1982) 'Chronic illness as biographical disruption', *Sociology of Health & Illness*, Vol. 4, No. 2, pp. 167–82

Byng-Hall, J. (1985) 'The family script: A useful bridge between theory and practice', *Journal of Family Therapy*, Vol. 7, No. 3, pp. 301–5

Cabinet Office and Social Exclusion Task Force (2007) *Reaching out: Think family. Analysis and Themes from the Families At Risk Review*, London: HMSO

Calman, K. and Hine, D. (1995) *A Policy Framework for Commissioning Cancer Services. A Report by the Expert Advisory Group on Cancer to the Chief Medical Officers of England and Wales*, London: Department of Health

Cancer Backup, Working with Cancer and Charted Institute of Personel and Development (2006) *Cancer and Working. Guidelines for Employers, HR and Line Managers*, London: Cancer Backup

Carers UK (2002) *Without Us? Calculating the Value of Carers' Support*, London: Carers UK

Cayless, S., Forbat, L., Illingworth, N., Hubbard, G. and Kearney, N. (2009) 'Men with prostate cancer over the first year of illness: Their experiences as biographical disruption', *Supportive Care in Cancer* (in press, Epub ahead of print: DOI 10-1007/s00520-009-0642-4)

Charmaz, K. (1983) 'Loss of self: a fundamental form of suffering in the chronically ill', *Sociology of Health & Illness*, Vol. 5, No. 2, pp. 168–95

Charmaz, K. (2004) 'Identity dilemmas of chronically ill men', *Sociological Quarterly*, Vol. 35, No. 2, pp. 269–88

Christiansen, C. H. (1999) 'Defining lives: Occupation as identity: An essay on competence, coherence, and the creation of meaning, The 1999 Eleanor Clarke Slagle Lecture', *American Journal of Occupational Therapy*, Vol. 53, No. 6, pp. 457–558

Corner, L. and Bond, J. (2004) 'Being at risk of dementia: Fears and anxieties of older adults', *Journal of Aging Studies*, Vol. 18, No. 2, pp. 143–155

Costain-Schou, K. and Hewison, J. (1999) *Facing Death – Experiencing Cancer*, Maidenhead: Open University Press

Cronen, V., Pearce, V. B. and Changsheng, X. (1989) 'The meaning of 'meaning' in the CMM analysis of communication: A comparison of two traditions', *Research on Language and Social Interaction*, Vol. 23, No. 1, pp. 1–40

Cancer Research UK (CRUK). 'UK Cancer Incidence Statistics' (online). Available from URL: http://info.cancerresearchuk.org/cancerstats/incidence/?a=5441 (accessed 24 March 2009)

Cutcliffe, J. R. (2003) 'Reconsidering reflexivity: introducing the case for intellectual entrepreneurship', *Qualitative Health Research*, Vol. 13, No. 1, pp. 136–48

Darzi, A. (2008) *High Quality Care for All. NHS Next Stage Review – Final Report*, London: Department of Health

Department of Health (2000) *The NHS Plan. A Plan for Investment. A Plan for Reform*, London: Department of Health

Department of Health (2001) *The Expert Patient: A New Approach to Chronic Disease management for the 21st century*, London: Department of Health

Department of Health (2005a) *Supporting People with Long Term Conditions. An NHS and Social Care Model to Support Local Innovation and Integration*, London: Department of Health

Department of Health (2005b) *Self Care – A Real Choice. Self Care Support – A Practical Option*, London: Department of Health

Department of Health (2006) *Our Health, our Care, our Say: Making it Happen*, London: Department of Health

Department of Health (2007) *Cancer Reform Strategy*, London: Department of Health

Dewey, J. (1963) *Experience and Education*, London: Collier and Macmillan

Epstein, D. (2008) *Down Under and Up Over: Travels with Narrative Therapy*, London: Karnac

Forbat, L. (2003) 'Relationship difficulties in dementia care. A discursive analysis of two women's accounts', *Dementia*, Vol. 2, No. 1, pp. 67–84

Forbat, L. (2005) *Talking about Care: Two Sides to the Story*, Bristol: Policy Press

Forbat, L. (2008) 'Social policy and relationship-centred dementia nursing', in Adams, T. (ed.) *Dementia Care Nursing*, Basingstoke: Palgrave/Macmillan, pp. 227–42

Forbat, L. and Henderson, J. (2003) '"Stuck in the middle with you": The ethics and process of qualitative research with two people in an intimate relationship', *Qualitative Health Research*, Vol. 13, No. 10, pp. 1453–62

Forbat, L. and Henderson, J. (2006) 'The professionalisation of informal carers?', in Davis, C. (ed.) *The Future Health Workforce*, Basingstoke: Palgrave Macmillan, pp. 49–67

Forbat, L. and Service, K. P. (2005) 'Who cares? Contextual layers in end-of-life care for people with intellectual disability and dementia', *Dementia*, Vol. 4, No. 3, pp. 413–31

Forbat, L., Hubbard, G. and Kearney, N. (2009) 'Patient and public involvement: models and muddles', *Journal of Clinical Nursing*, Jan 8 (Epub ahead of print)

Foucault, M. (1977) *Discipline and Punish*, London: Penguin

Foucault, M. (2006) *The Birth of the Clinic*, London: Routledge

Fu, M. R., LeMone, P. and McDaniel, R. W. (2004) 'An integrated approach to an anlysis of symptom management in patients with cancer', *Oncology Nursing Forum*, Vol. 31, No. 1, pp. 65–70

Gershenson Hodgson, L., Cutler, S. and Livingston, K. (1999) 'Alzheimer's disease and symptom-seeking', *American Journal of Alzheimer's Disease and Other Dementias*, Vol. 14, No. 6, pp. 364–74

Goffman, E. (1963) *Stigma: Notes on the Management of Spoiled Identity*, New Jersey: Prentice-Hall

Greer, S. L. and Rowland, D. (2008) *Devolving Policy, Diverging Values? The Values of the United Kingdom's National Health Services*, London: The Nuffield Trust

Gregory, S. (2005) 'Living with chronic illness in the family setting', *Sociology of Health and Illness*, Vol. 27, No. 3, pp. 372–92

Halldórsdóttir, S. and Hamrin, E. (1996) 'Experiencing existential changes: the lived experience of having cancer', *Cancer Nursing*, Vol. 19, No. 1, pp. 29–36

Henderson, J. and Forbat, L. (2002) 'Relationship-based social policy: personal and policy constructions of "care"', *Critical Social Policy*, Vol. 22, No. 4, pp. 669–87

Hubbard, G., Kidd, L., Donaghy, E., McDonald, C. and Kearney, N. (2007) 'A review of literature about involving people affected by cancer in research, policy and planning and practice', *Patient Education and Counseling*, Vol. 65, No. 1, pp. 21–33

Hubbard, G., Kidd, L. and Kearney, N. (2009a) 'Disrupted lives and threats to identity: The experiences of people with colorectal cancer within the first year following diagnosis', *Health*, in press

Hubbard, G., Illingworth, N., Rowa-Dewar, N., Forbat, L. and Kearney, N. (2009b) 'Treatment decision making in cancer care: The role of the carer', *Journal of Clinical Nursing*, in press

Illingworth, N., Forbat, L., Hubbard, G. and Kearney, N. (2009) 'The importance of relationships in the experience of cancer: a re-working of the policy ideal of whole-systems working', *European Journal of Oncology Nursing*, in press

Information Service Division (ISD) (2006) *SPARRA: Scottish Patients at Risk of Readmission and Admission*, Edinburgh: NHS; National Services Scotland

Johnston, B. (2005) 'Editorial How does the media portray cancer?', *International Journal of Palliative Nursing*, Vol. 11, No. 10, pp. 5–8

Kennedy, F., Haslam, C., Munir, F. and Pryce, J. (2007) 'Returning to work following cancer: a qualitative exploratory study into the experience of returning to work following cancer', *European Journal of Cancer Care*, Vol. 16, No. 1, pp. 17–25

Kim, Y., Baker, F., Spollers, R. L. and Wellisch, D. (2006) 'Psychological adjustment of cancer caregivers with multiple roles', *Psycho-oncology*, Vol. 15, No. 9, pp. 795–804

Kolb, D. A. (1984) *Experiential Learning: Experience as the Source of Learning and Development*, Englewood Cliffs: Prentice Hall

Lacasse, C. B. and Beck, S. L. (2007) 'Clinical assessment of symptom clusters', *Seminars in Oncology Nursing*, Vol. 23, No. 2, pp. 106–12

Lambert, M. and Barley, D. (2001). 'Research summary on the therapeutic relationship and psychotherapy outcome', *Psychotherapy: Theory, Research, Practice, Training*, Vol. 38, No. 4, pp. 357–61

Lee, V. (2008) 'The existential plight of cancer: meaning making as a concrete approach to the intangible search for meaning', *Supportive Care in Cancer*, Vol. 16, No. 7, pp. 779–85

Lorig, K. (2002) 'Partnership between expert patients and physicians', *Lancet*, Vol. 9309, No. 359, pp. 814–15

Main, D. S., Nowells, C. T., Cavender, T. A., Etschmaier, M. and Steiner, J. F. (2005) 'A qualitative study of work and work return in cancer survivors', *Psycho-oncology*, Vol. 14, No. 11, pp. 992–1004

Maunsell, E., Drolet, M., Brisson, J., Brisson, C., Masse, B. and Deschenes, L. (2004) 'Work situation after breast cancer: Results from a population based study', *Journal of the National Cancer Institute*, Vol. 96, No. 24, pp. 1813–22

Montgomery, E. (2004) 'Tortured families: A coordinated management of meaning analysis', *Family Process*, Vol. 4, No. 3, pp. 349–71

Morris, S. M. (2001) 'Joint and individual interviewing in the context of cancer', *Qualitative Health Research*, Vol. 11, No. 4, pp. 553–67

Mulders, M., Vingershoets, A. and Breed, V. (2008) 'The impact of cancer and chemotherapy – Perceptual similarities and differences between cancer patients, nurses and physicians', *European Journal of Oncology Nursing*, Vol. 12, No. 2, pp. 97–102

NHS Quality Improvement Scotland (QIS) (2007) *Cancer Services – Draft Core Standards. April 2007*, Edinburgh: NHS Quality Improvement Scotland

National Institute for Health and Clinical Excellence (NICE) (2004) *Improving Supportive and Palliative Care for Adults with Cancer*, NICE, London

Office for Public Management (OPM), Care21 and Scottish Executive (2006) *The Future of Unpaid Care in Scotland*, Edinburgh: Scottish Executive

Robb, M. and Forbat, L. (2005) 'Introduction', in Malone, C., Forbat, L., Robb, M. and Seden, J (eds) *Relating Experience: Stories from Health and Social Care*, London: Routledge, pp. 1–3

Rolland, J. S. (1994) *Families, Illness and Disability: An Integrative Treatment Model*, New York: Basic Books

Rolland, J. S. (1999) 'Parental Illness and Disability', *Journal of Family Therapy*, Vol. 21, No. 3, pp. 242–66

Schon, D. (1983) *The Reflective Practitioner: How Professionals Think in Action*, London: Harper Collins

Scottish Executive (2001a) *Cancer in Scotland: Action for Change*, Edinburgh: Scottish Executive

Scottish Executive (2001b) *Cancer in Scotland: Action for Change. A Guide to Securing Access to Information*, Edinburgh: Scottish Executive

Scottish Executive (2003) *Partnership for Care: Scotland's Health White Paper*, Edinburgh: Scottish Executive

Scottish Executive (2004) *Cancer in Scotland. Sustaining Change*, Edinburgh: Scottish Executive

Scottish Executive (2005a) *A National Framework for Service Change in the NHS in Scotland. Building a Health Service Fit for the Future. Volume 2: A guide for the NHS*, Edinburgh: Scottish Executive

Scottish Executive (2005b) *Delivering for Health*, Edinburgh: Scottish Executive

Scottish Executive (2005c) *A National Framework for Service Change in the NHS in Scotland. Building a Health Service Fit for the Future. Summary*, Edinburgh: Scottish Executive

Scottish Executive (2005d) *Building a Health Service Fit for the Future.* Edinburgh: Scottish Executive

Scottish Executive (2006a) *Delivering Care, Enabling Health*, Edinburgh: Scottish Executive

Scottish Executive (2006b) *Visible, Accessible and Integrated Care. Report of the Review of Nursing in the Community in Scotland*, Edinburgh: Scottish Executive

Scottish Executive (2007) *Co-ordinated, Integrated and Fit for Purpose*, Edinburgh: Scottish Executive

Scottish Executive Health Department (2002) Community Care and Health (Scotland) Act 2002, London: OPSI

Scottish Government (2005) Smoking, Health and Social Care (Scotland) Act 2005, London: OPSI

Scottish Government (2008) *Better Cancer Care*, Edinburgh: Scottish Government

Scottish Government (2009) 'Shifting the balance of care' (online). Available from URL: www.shiftingthebalance.scot.nhs.uk/ (accessed 8 April 2009)

Sherman, A. and Simonton, S. (1999) 'Family therapy for cancer patients: Clinical issues and interventions', *The Family Journal of Counselling and Therapy for Couples and Families*, Vol. 7, No. 1, pp. 39–50

Shilling, V., Jenkins, V. and Fallowfield, L. J. (2003) 'Factors affecting patient and clinician satisfaction with the clinical consultation: Can communication skills training for clinicians improve satisfaction?', *Psycho-oncology*, Vol. 12, No. 6, pp. 599–611

Sitzia, J., Cotterell, P. and Richardson, A. (2004) *Formative Evaluation of the Cancer Partnership Project*, London: Macmillan Cancer Relief

Spelten, E. R., Sprangers, M. A. G. and Verbeek, J. H. O. M. (2002) 'Factors reported to influence the return to work of cancer survivors: A literature review', *Psycho-oncology*, Vol. 11, No. 2, pp. 124–31

Steiner, J. F., Cavender, T. A., Main, D. S. and Bradley, C. J. (2007) 'Assessing the impact of cancer on work outcomes', *Cancer*, Vol. 101, No. 8, pp. 1703–11

Verdecchia, A., Francisci, S., Brenner, H., Gatta, G., Micheli, A., Mangone, L. and Kunkler, I. (2007) 'Recent cancer survival in Europe: a 2000-02 period analysis of EUROCARE-4 data', *Lancet Oncology*, Vol. 8, No. 9, pp. 784–96

Vinkopur, A. D. and Vinkopur-Kaplan, D. (1990) 'In sickness and in health. Patterns of social support and undermining in older married couples', *Journal of Aging and Health*, Vol. 2, No. 2, pp. 215–41

Vos, M. S. and de Haes, J. (2007) 'Denial in cancer patients, an explorative review', *Psycho-oncology*, Vol. 16, No. 1, pp. 12–25

Weisman, A. D. and Worden, J. W. (1976) 'The existential plight in cancer: significance of the first 100 days', *International Journal of Psychiatry Medicine*, Vol. 7, No. 1, pp. 1–15

Index